1991

Information Systems for Ambulatory Care

Edited by Theodore A. Matson
Division of Ambulatory Care and Health Promotion of the American Hospital Association

and Mark D. McDougall
Sheldon I. Dorenfest & Associates, Ltd.

American Hospital Publishing, Inc.,
a wholly owned subsidiary of the
American Hospital Association

The views expressed in this publication are strictly those of the authors and do not necessarily represent official positions of the American Hospital Association.

Library of Congress Cataloging-in-Publication Data

Information systems for ambulatory care / edited by Theodore A. Matson
    and Mark D. McDougall.
       p.   cm.
    Includes bibliographical references.
    ISBN 1-55648-048-2
    1. Ambulatory medical care—Data processing. 2. Information
storage and retrieval systems—Ambulatory medical care. I. Matson,
Theodore A. II. McDougall, Mark D.
RA409.5.I53   1990
362.1'2'0285—dc20   90-189
                                         CIP

Catalog no. 093100

©1990 by American Hospital Publishing, Inc.,
a wholly owned subsidiary of the
American Hospital Association

Printed in the USA

ᗩᕼᗩ is a service mark of the American Hospital Association used under license by American Hospital Publishing, Inc.

Text set in Palatino
2.5M—05/90—0258

Linda Conheady, Richard Hill, Project Editors
Sophie Yarborough, Editorial Assistant
Marcia Bottoms, Managing Editor
Peggy DuMais, Production Coordinator
Marcia Vecchione, Designer
Brian Schenk, Books Division Director

Cover photograph courtesy of H. Armstrong Roberts, Inc., Philadelphia.

Contents

Part One.   Key Considerations

List of Figures

List of Tables

Contributors

Raymond D. Aller, M.D., is director, Medical Group Pathology Laboratory, Santa Barbara, California, and is also medical director, Tri-Counties Blood Bank; pathologist, Santa Barbara Cottage Hospital, and director of laboratory, Santa Ynez Valley Hospital, Solvang, California. He is associate clinical professor of pathology, University of Southern California School of Medicine. He serves as contributing editor of *CAP Today,* the official publication of the College of American Pathologists.

Margret K. Amatayakul, R.R.A., M.B.A., is associate executive director, American Medical Record Association, Chicago, Illinois. She was previously associate professor, Department of Medical Record Administration, at the University of Illinois Medical Center.

Jill Crowell, Ph.D., is president, Crowell and Associates, Seattle, Washington, which consults with health and human services organizations in management and information systems planning and implementation. Her previous experience includes serving as vice-president for information systems, Pacific Medical Center, Seattle, and managing the development and test site for PHAMIS, Inc.'s patient care system, The Last Word. She has also managed the development of claims processing and referral management systems for a large HMO and the development and implementation of systems for national and state health care agencies. In addition to other academic appointments, she was an international exchange faculty in management and information systems at West China University of Medical Sciences in Chengdu, Sichuan Province, People's Republic of China.

Erica L. Drazen, M.A., is vice-president and director of the health care practice of Arthur D. Little, Inc. For the past 20 years, the focus of her practice has been on research and consulting in health care information systems. She has performed research on diffusion and use of computerized ECG analysis, computerized monitoring, patient appointment scheduling, bedside terminals, and automated medical records. Her consulting practice is focused on developing information systems plans to organizational strategies and, as appropriate, applications of new technologies. She has worked for hospitals, hospital systems, and ambulatory care practices. Mrs. Drazen is a doctoral candidate at the Harvard School of Public Health, where she is conducting research on physician acceptance of computers. She is an active member of the Healthcare Information Management Systems Society of the American Hospital Association and is current chairman of the Center for Healthcare Information Management.

Robert J. Feldman, M.E., is vice-president of Sneider & Associates, Newton, Massachusetts, a health care consulting firm specializing in information systems and operations management. Mr. Feldman has assisted health care institutions in over 25 states and provinces to improve current systems or to acquire and implement new systems. His previous associations include Sheldon I. Dorenfest & Associates, VHA Enterprises, Technicon Data Systems, and Medical College of Virginia Hospitals.

Ronald L. Gue, Ph.D., is president, Phoenix Medical Systems, Inc., Gaithersburg, Maryland, a startup company that focuses on software and services to support implementation of major health care information systems. Prior to forming Phoenix, Dr. Gue was executive vice-president of Sheldon I. Dorenfest & Associates, Ltd., an information systems consulting firm specializing in health care. Dr. Gue has held a number of academic and business positions during his 30 years in the health care information systems industry. These include founder and first chairman and president of The Medicus Corporation; chairman, Computer Sciences Department, Southern Methodist University; and national director, Healthcare Services, Arthur Young & Company.

Helen L. Hill is director of data management, MEDSTAT Systems, Inc., Ann Arbor, Michigan, a health care cost-containment information systems firm. At the time of this book, she was a senior consultant with Sheldon I. Dorenfest & Associates, Ltd., Chicago, Illinois, an information systems consulting firm specializing in health care. Prior to this, she was responsible for systems planning and development at Catherine McAuley Health Center, Ann Arbor, Michigan. Ms. Hill has more than 20 years' experience in information systems. She specializes in strategic and tactical planning, vendor evaluation and selection, systems implementation management, systems development, and consulting. She has published several articles on health care information systems.

Matthew Kelliher, M.B.A, is director of operations design and engineering at Harvard Community Health Plan, Brookline, Massachusetts. His responsibilities include providing systems, quality, and operations improvement expertise to Harvard Health's network of health centers, medical groups, hospital affiliates, and corporate management offices. His past experience includes serving in systems-related staff and consulting roles at the University of California, San Diego; Medicus Systems Corporation; and several East Coast teaching hospitals.

O. John Kralovec is a practice director with First Consulting Group, Long Beach, California, and a nationally recognized leader in the field of information systems benefits realization. Mr. Kralovec's work with Stanford University Hospital resulted in the leading methodology for identifying and achieving tangible clinical and operational benefits from information systems. His extensive experience in information systems, operations/ productivity enhancement and quality improvement has resulted in a unique and highly successful approach to benefits realization. For fifteen years, Mr. Kralovec has been consulting to a wide variety of health care organizations including independent not-for-profit facilities, international multifacility corporations, and numerous internationally recognized academic medical centers. Mr. Kralovec is a frequent speaker and the author of numerous articles on health care information systems, systems benefits realization, operations/ productivity enhancement, and quality improvement.

Elody F. Krieger is coordinator, physician information services, Columbus Children's Hospital, Columbus, Ohio. Her current responsibilities include providing development and ongoing maintenance of the Children's Hospital Link, an electronic link between Children's Hospital and its community physicians; serving as information services liaison to the medical staff; and serving as computer consultant to private practice physicians. Her other relevant experience includes implementing an information center at Grant Medical Center, Columbus. She has over 12 years' experience in the use of computing technologies in a medical environment.

Ellen Marszalek-Gaucher, M.S., is senior associate director, University of Michigan Hospitals, Ann Arbor, Michigan. She manages the operation of an 888-bed hospital with 32,000 admissions per year and 780,000 outpatient clinic visits. She serves on the editorial board of *Health Care Competition* newsletter and the executive committee of the National Demonstration Project on Quality funded by the Hartford Foundation and the Harvard Community Health Plan. She is a member of the American College for Health Care Executives and a charter member of the Society of Ambulatory Care Professionals. She is coauthoring a book called *Transforming Healthcare Organizations* for Jossey-Bass Publishers. Previously she was the associate director of ambulatory care and played a major role in the design and activation of the A. Alfred Taubman Center, a 300,000-square-foot ambulatory care center. She also developed plans and implemented a satellite network of six comprehensive primary care centers and three specialty clinics.

Gerald R. Mathys, M.B.A., is executive vice-president, Sheldon I. Dorenfest & Associates, Ltd., Chicago, Illinois, an information systems consulting firm specializing in health care. His previous experience includes serving as president of Sentry Data, Inc., as general manager of Technicon Medical Information Systems, and as midwest regional manager of Shared Medical Systems. He has over 20 years of experience in health care systems development and implementation and has frequently spoken before several professional groups, including the Healthcare Financial Management Association (HFMA), the Healthcare Information and Management Systems Society (HIMSS), and the American Hospital Association.

Theodore A. Matson, M.A., is senior staff specialist, Division of Ambulatory Care and Health Promotion, American Hospital Association, Chicago, Illinois. In this capacity, he is responsible for providing strategic direction and consultation to the health care industry in the areas of hospital-based ambulatory care services, ambulatory surgery, freestanding ambulatory care facilities, emergency medical services, and ambulatory care information systems. In addition, he provides representation and advocacy services and participates in public policy developments regarding ambulatory care issues. Mr. Matson is a national and international speaker in ambulatory care. He serves as editor of the American Hospital Association's publication *Outreach*, the sole industry resource devoted exclusively to hospital perspectives on ambulatory care issues. A frequent writer on ambulatory care topics, he is also the editor of *The Hospital Emergency Department: Returning to Financial Viability*, and *Restructuring for Ambulatory Care: A Guide to Reorganization* published by American Hospital Publishing, Inc.

Mark D. McDougall is senior consultant, Sheldon I. Dorenfest & Associates, Ltd., Chicago, Illinois, an information systems consulting firm specializing in health care. Mr. McDougall assists hospitals to develop and implement improved automation strategies such that the benefits of automation are realized. He was formerly associate director, Healthcare Information and Management Systems Society (HIMSS) and was the past president of the HIMSS Greater Chicago chapter. He is now a senior member with the HIMSS. His prior experience includes conducting productivity improvement studies as a management consultant with the Chicago Hospital Council and later as a management engineer with Evangelical Health Systems, Oak Brook, Illinois. He has recently coedited another AHPI publication entitled *Productivity and Performance Management in Health Care Institutions* (Chicago: American Hospital Publishing, 1989).

Lisa Osteraas was formerly systems engineer at Harvard Community Health Plan, Brookline, Massachusetts. Her past experience includes systems consulting at Norton Company in Worcester, Massachusetts. She is a member of the Healthcare Information and Management Systems Society (HIMSS) and the Institute of Industrial Engineers.

Margaret D. Sabin, MHSA, is administrator, Medical Centers of Colorado, a family practice and occupational medicine network under ownership of Lutheran Medical Center, Wheatridge, Colorado. She previously was director of management services at Denver Health and Hospitals, Denver, Colorado. She serves on the board of directors for the Society for Ambulatory Care Professionals and is the vice-president for the Colorado chapter of the Healthcare Financial Management Association.

Thomas A. Stocker, M.B.A., is director, information systems development, Lutheran Medical Center, Denver, Colorado. He is currently investigating systems incorporating integrated functions within an extensive provider network. His prior experience includes directing the MIS function at a large hospital and consulting with a big-8 accounting firm. Mr. Stocker is the current president of the Colorado chapter of the Healthcare Information and Management Systems Society and a member of the Coopers E. Lybrand CIO Forum.

Lawrence D. Visk, M.B.A., is senior consultant, Sheldon I. Dorenfest & Associates, Ltd., Chicago, Illinois, an information systems consulting firm specializing in health care. At Dorenfest he has performed a systems assessment of the Michigan Health Care Network and has been involved with several selection and implementation engagements of ambulatory care systems. Mr. Visk was previously with HBO and Company, where he served as manager of the Midwest division advanced products and technical support, and as installation manager.

Walter C. Zerrenner, M.A., is vice-president, information services, and chief information officer, Methodist Hospital of Indiana, Inc., Indianapolis, Indiana. Methodist is a 1,200-bed tertiary care teaching hospital with extensive health care networks throughout the greater Indianapolis area. The hospital is nationally renowned for its organ transplant program and its emergency medicine and trauma center. Mr. Zerrenner's previous experience includes serving as vice-president, information systems, Evangelical Health Systems, Oak Brook, Illinois. This multihospital regional health care system manages five hospitals and an extensive

managed care network in a seven-county region in the Chicago area.
At Evangelical Systems, Mr. Zerrenner was responsible for the five-year
plan for the information systems and the selection and implementation
of an open communication architecture to support the complex managed
care network. His other positions have included regional manager at
Value Computing, Inc.; corporate director, information systems, at NCR;
manager, information systems at Borden, Inc.; systems consultant at CBS,
Inc., and president of his own consulting practice.

Preface

An unprecedented level of changes in the health care industry has resulted in considerable turmoil for our nation's health care providers, suppliers, and patients. The most pressing of all challenges facing our institutions is continuing to deliver high-quality care while responding effectively to the cost pressures being exerted upon our hospitals and medical professionals.

In order to address this challenge, hospitals are searching for more efficient ways to manage costs. Among the available alternatives, the effective use of automation to manage and access critical information is proving to be a strategic tool in the containment of costs. Better hospital management requires better automation. Effective information systems are especially important in ambulatory care, where multiple providers treat patients in various settings.

As ambulatory care growth has proliferated, so have the requests for automating the outpatient environment. In early 1988, the Division of Ambulatory Care of the American Hospital Association began advising health care providers as they sought to develop and enhance their information systems for ambulatory care needs. Subsequently, one of the first nationwide attempts to provide the health care industry with insight into these needs was a two-day seminar held in June 1988. It was co-sponsored by two American Hospital Association societies, the Healthcare Information and Management Systems Society (HIMSS) and the Society for Ambulatory Care Professionals (SACP). This seminar, entitled "Information Systems for Ambulatory Care," was very successful and later repeated. With the magnitude of requests for consultation increasing, and recognizing the obvious high level of interest and need for helpful guidelines for automating the ambulatory care arena, we embarked on this publishing effort.

Although this book may not answer all of your questions, it was developed to provide you with a better understanding of the key issues that influence effective computer use in ambulatory care. The book will assist in meeting the planning, organizational, and managerial challenges of health care organizations undergoing the automation of ambulatory care service delivery.

When developing strategies for improving the effectiveness of automation programs, several issues that require attention are important regardless of the type of information system under consideration for purchase or replacement. Examples of such issues that are relevant to any automation improvement effort include:

- Identifying opportunities for improving management through automation
- Objectively assessing automation needs and examining strategic options
- Evaluating systems and developing practical implementation strategies
- Planning for and conducting benefit realization efforts

Therefore, while still very relevant to ambulatory care information systems programs, portions of this book are more generic in nature and applicable to all types of automation programs.

The book is organized into two sections. The first section begins with an overview (chapter 1), discusses macro and micro perspectives on the ambulatory care environment (chapter 2), and covers current ambulatory care information systems and new technologies (chapter 3). Chapters 4 through 7 provide a framework for determining information systems needs, implementing a system, and realizing benefits. Chapter 8 discusses how changing methods of payment for ambulatory care services will affect delivery of those services. The last part of the section reviews the marketplace and profiles vendors who are among the market leaders in ambulatory care software and hardware (chapter 9).

In part 2, chapters 10 to 16 provide general overviews of issues pertinent to various ambulatory care settings and enumerate the specific information requirements for ambulatory surgery, the emergency and radiology departments, medical records, clinical laboratories, multiple freestanding ambulatory care centers, and referral management systems. The last three chapters offer widely applicable examples drawn from specific institutions. These chapters deal with appointment scheduling, outpatient clinics, and physician office systems.

The book concludes with two appendixes: one lists approximately 140 software vendors that offer ambulatory care related products, and the other lists appointment scheduling vendors. In addition, the annotated bibliography includes literature on such topics as system implementation and evaluation, benefits of computerization, and cost-accounting and decision support systems.

We would like to thank the contributing authors for their willingness to partake in this endeavor and share their expertise with the field. Thanks also to Cheryl Allen, secretary in the Division of Ambulatory Care, for her help in typing the manuscripts; Ed Zimmerman, research assistant, Division of Ambulatory Care, for his invaluable research efforts; Linda Conheady, assistant managing editor, American Hospital Publishing, Inc., for her editorial guidance during the production phase; Sophie Yarborough, editorial assistant, AHPI, for assuming day-to-day backup to ensure orderly flow of the editing process; and Brian Schenk, vice-president, Books Division, AHPI, for his leadership in publishing widely acclaimed texts on ambulatory care service delivery.

We are hopeful that this book will provide readers with many useful strategies for improving results from their investments in computerization.

Mark D. McDougall
Theodore A. Matson

Part One

Key Considerations

Chapter 1

Introduction and Overview

Mark D. McDougall and Theodore A. Matson

The challenges posed by today's changing health care environment—increased competition, declining use of hospital inpatient facilities, prospective reimbursement legislation, and the changing roles of private industry and insurers—make it imperative for hospitals to realize more fully the potential benefits of automation.[1] Computerization provides unparalleled opportunities for hospitals to improve operational efficiency and effectiveness, particularly in ambulatory care.

There can be little argument that the federal prospective payment system environment brought with it some of the most fundamental and far-reaching changes that the United States health care marketplace has ever experienced. It has changed the way business is done. It has changed how decisions are made both from a business point of view as well as clinically. It has even changed some of the approaches to the practice of medicine, with its continuing emphasis on substituting inpatient care for ambulatory care. Most certainly it has changed the amount and kind of information required to manage and operate today's health care organizations, which has resulted in the need for structural changes in the information systems that support the decision-making process in these institutions.[2] We have, most probably, only seen the beginning of these changes.

Although ambulatory care has received moderate attention relative to inpatient care, many underestimate the long-term impact this segment of health care will have in the future. The shift from inpatient to outpatient care is evidenced by the following:

- Ambulatory care is now the only growth segment among the current hospital-based services.
- The number of hospital outpatient visits exceeds the number of acute care days on a nationwide basis.

- Total hospital revenues from outpatient care grew from 12 percent in 1983 to 26 percent in 1988, a 117 percent increase.[3]
- It is predicted that by 1995 a majority of hospitals will derive 50 percent of their revenue from outpatient businesses.[4]
- The number of freestanding ambulatory care providers is projected to double from 1980 to 1990, while the number of hospital-based providers will drop slightly (table 1-1).

This movement toward outpatient services will create great challenges for hospitals to manage the unique operational and clinical needs of ambulatory care service delivery. The information system that is required to service an institution in this kind of environment is one that provides efficiency of operations and flexibility. It must be efficient in the sense that it is easy to use, easy to change, and relatively easy to program for new system requirements. If it is able to meet these efficiency criteria, it will also provide the flexibility that is required.

To the extent that a system provides these characteristics to the user, it provides a competitive advantage over the organization that has an information system without these characteristics. A system with these features will not guarantee success to the organization, but it will certainly improve the probabilities for success.[5] Implementing information systems can result in better work-load scheduling, improved patient flow and processing, enhanced scope of information captured, increased accuracy of information, reduction in the number of employees, and many other benefits.

The Importance of Information Management

Health care is clearly an information-intensive industry. Hospitals need information to make crucial decisions affecting both the clinical course of patients and the strategic course of the institution. Nonetheless, as compared to other industries health care has generally underinvested in information management.[6] Although health care is somewhere between manufacturing and banking in *information intensity*, information systems spending in the health care industry lags considerably

Table 1-1. Number of Ambulatory Care Providers, 1970–1990

Ambulatory Care Provider Type	1970	1980	1990 (Est.)
Freestanding	7,892	19,516	39,550
Hospital-based	5,859	5,904	5,600

Source: Division of Ambulatory Care, American Hospital Association, 1989.

behind the others (table 1-2). The use of the term *information intensity* as used here is subjective, but it does indicate the relative value of the computerized information in the various industries.

Historically, health care information systems have been used to collect, store, and retrieve *data*.

So far, most computer users still apply the new technology only to do faster what they have always done before, to crunch conventional numbers. However, as soon as a company takes the first tentative steps from individual data elements to meaningful information, its decision processes, management structure, and even the way its work gets done begin to be significantly enhanced. *Information* is data endowed with relevance and purpose.[7]

Although mountains of reports with tremendous amounts of data are often generated, they usually do not provide hospital management with the *information* needed to make well-informed strategic decisions to curtail costs, increase revenues, and enhance quality of care. Therefore, hospital management needs to harness their information systems in such a way that they have ongoing access to the precious information needed to develop and maintain a sustainable competitive advantage. For ambulatory care, this entails tracking the flow of patients through various departments, documenting the amount and types of resources expended, assigning costs and charges at individual procedural and case-specific levels, and reporting these events by unique patient profiles.

Another example of data being translated into meaningful information pertains to hospitals negotiating beneficial contracts with health maintenance organizations (HMOs) and preferred provider organizations (PPOs). Most patient accounting systems generate total patient changes by payer type for a given period. However, contracts with HMOs and PPOs are usually based on per diems. Therefore, in preparation of HMO/PPO contract negotiations, hospitals need to monitor and analyze (at a minimum) the billing data by payer type (including the HMOs and PPOs) and determine the per diem average and variance. Of course, much more information is needed to negotiate successful contracts. Nonetheless, this example illustrates the difference between data (that

Table 1-2. Information Intensity and Information Systems Spending by Industry

Variable	Industry		
	Manufacturing	**Health**	**Banking**
Information intensity index	30	40	60
Information systems spending as percentage of total expenditures	5%	2.6%	7%

Source: American Hospital Association. *Guide to Effective Health Care Information Management and the Role of the Chief Information Officer.* Chicago: American Hospital Association, 1988, pp. 3, 21.

is, total patient charges) and meaningful information (per diem average and variance).

Expectations for Information Systems

Over the years, many organizations have purchased and installed information systems with the expectation that significant benefits would accrue. As John Kralovec points out in chapter 7, it was often found that once systems were installed, benefits and anticipated savings never materialized, and in some cases system-related expenditures actually increased. Achieving benefits from information systems has become not only an economic necessity but, for many institutions, a critical factor in the difference between success or failure. This will be an even greater challenge for systems devoted to ambulatory care needs, for their development has significantly lagged behind the investments and attention given to inpatient systems.

As costs for information systems continue to rise, hospital management is increasingly concerned that these systems be cost-justified. Senior health care executives are now being held accountable for demonstrating a tangible financial return on the investment in information systems. Detailed cost justification has become an essential part of the entire system selection decision-making process—a trend that will no doubt continue.

Information systems are also expected to provide for improved operational control. The information systems vendors that will be most successful in the future are the ones who demonstrate they can assist hospitals in optimizing productivity levels, streamlining day-to-day operations, and enhancing quality of service.

Substantial Expense, Unmet Needs

Even though health care still lags considerably behind other industries in information systems spending as a percentage of total expenditures, health care's total expenditures for computer-related products and services are staggering (figure 1-1).

Despite this substantial investment in automation, many hospital computer needs remain unmet. Hospital computer systems are failing to fulfill their potential because of various feature deficiencies, shortcomings in installation methods and postinstallation support, exaggerations of product capabilities by vendors, and the difficulties of integrating systems. Many products billed as integrated systems simply do not work, while others do not provide enough functionality.[8] These factors have led to a slowdown in the rate of growth in hospital expenditures for computer-related products and services (table 1-3).

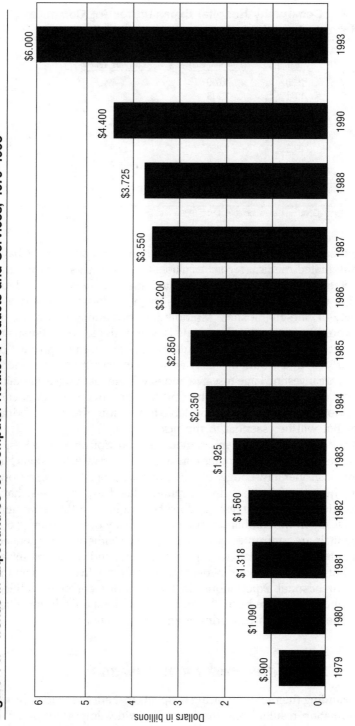

Figure 1-1. Trends in Expenditures for Computer-Related Products and Services, 1979–1993

Year	Dollars in billions
1979	$.900
1980	$1.090
1981	$1.318
1982	$1.560
1983	$1.925
1984	$2.350
1985	$2.850
1986	$3.200
1987	$3.550
1988	$3.725
1990	$4.400
1993	$6.000

Source: Copyright ©1989 by Sheldon I. Dorenfest & Associates, Ltd.

Table 1-3.   Community Hospital Expenditures for Computer-Related Products and Services

Year	Total ($ in millions)	% Growth over Previous Year
1980	1,090	—
1981	1,318	20.9
1982	1,560	18.4
1983	1,925	23.4
1984	2,350	22.1
1985	2,850	21.3
1986	3,200	12.3
1987	3,550	10.9
1988	3,725	4.9

Source: Sheldon I. Dorenfest & Associates, Ltd., 1989.

The ideal hospital information system that is needed would have a fully automated medical record available for all patients showing the history of all treatments. This automated medical record would be accessed or updated by authorized users, such as physicians or nurses, at a variety of care-giving sites. Multiple files containing similar information would be automatically updated using a single entry. Financial and cost-accounting information would be collected as a by-product of the care process and would be easily available to users.[9] Unfortunately, as vendors are investing large research and development budgets in maintaining and modestly expanding their present product lines, it appears that they do not have the funds available to invest in the new product function that will be essential in the next decade.

As hospitals have become much more cost-conscious, the time hospitals consume for making computer hardware and software decisions has lengthened considerably. Longer buying processes, together with a slowdown in the rate of increase in computer-related expenditures, have begun to affect even the largest vendors' bottom line. In this extremely competitive environment many vendors continually oversell their products. Hospitals are confronted with questionable claims and exaggerated capabilities by system vendors. Competition is fierce and vendor promises escalate, but performance and benefits usually do not live up to vendor promises or hospital expectations. In this environment of unfulfilled promises, hospitals have been "burned" and understandably have become a little gun-shy in procuring information systems.

Interim Solutions and Future Needs

Notwithstanding the problems facing hospitals that are trying to improve their automation results, computerization provides important benefits to hospitals today. Knowing that the fully integrated hospital information systems they seek will not be developed for some time, hospitals are acknowledging that many products they are currently buying are only interim solutions. They are scaling their expectations down to a more realistic level. Although products being purchased now may have built-in obsolescence, they nonetheless represent progress in hospitals' approaches to automation. Hospitals continue to learn to utilize today's computer technology more efficiently and effectively as they await the fully integrated comprehensive information systems of the future.

Conclusion

Because the future of ambulatory care will include multiple providers in very diverse settings, a hospital's ability to link various systems (for example, clinical, financial, operations, management) into a continuum of care may ultimately determine its survival or failure. With ambulatory care revenues projected to represent nearly half of total hospital revenues by the mid-1990s, the integration and reporting of accurate, timely data for ambulatory care will no doubt be one of the highest priorities of each institution in this decade.

References

1. Sheldon I. Dorenfest & Associates, Ltd. *Hospital Information Systems: State of the Art.* 1988 ed. Northbrook, IL: SID, 1988, p. 1.

2. Schmitz, H. H. *Managing Health Care Information Resources.* Rockville, MD: Aspen Publishers, Inc., 1987, pp. 78–79.

3. American Hospital Association. *Hospital Statistics.* 1984 and 1989 editions. Chicago: AHA, 1984 and 1989.

4. Matson, T. A. Rethinking the delivery of ambulatory care: hospital-based vs. freestanding alternatives. Presentation, Penetrating the Alternate Site Marketplace Conference, Biomedical Business International, San Francisco, Sept. 15, 1987.

5. Schmitz, p. 95.

6. American Hospital Association. *Guide to Effective Health Care Information Management and the Role of the Chief Information Officer.* Chicago: AHA, 1988, pp. 1–3.

7. Drucker, P. F. The coming of the new organization. *Harvard Business Review* 66(1):45–53, Jan.–Feb. 1988.

8. Sheldon I. Dorenfest, pp. 271–72.

9. Dorenfest, S. I. Healthcare forecast: lessons of the '80s give way to challenges of the '90s. *HealthWeek* 3(25):33, Dec. 18, 1989.

Chapter 2

The Ambulatory Care Environment

Theodore A. Matson

The first part of this chapter briefly reviews the shift from acute care to ambulatory care, discusses settings where ambulatory care is provided, and describes specific programs and services. The second part describes challenges in the health care environment that will affect ambulatory care information systems in the future.

From Acute Care to Ambulatory Care

The provision of acute care in hospitals historically has led to systems being built primarily for inpatients. Admissions, patient days, length of stay, "product lines," and "centers of excellence" all reflect the emphasis that inpatient services have received. Because of this orientation, information systems developments have also occurred for the exclusivity of inpatient care needs.

Unfortunately, the acute care hospital industry in the 1990s is characterized as a matured marketplace. Marketplace incentives such as the Medicare prospective payment system, utilization review, managed care, and alternative providers have lessened the once-dominant provider of multidimensional hospital and health care services. *Ambulatory care,* the provision of health care services to patients who do not remain in a hospital overnight, is now emerging as the key point of health care delivery.[1]

As the hospital industry continues to evolve, it is conceivable that ambulatory care development and expansion will continue for the next two to three decades. In terms of information systems requirements, the capture and reporting of key data elements associated with each ambulatory care visit will be critical to measure productivity and ensure efficiency in managing patient care.

To understand the complexity of the evolving ambulatory care marketplace, it is important to illustrate the provision of services from both macro and micro perspectives.

A Macro Perspective on Ambulatory Care

Because ambulatory care refers to the provision of services provided to patients who are not hospitalized, any service provided to a patient on a less-than-24-hour basis can be considered an ambulatory visit.

Ambulatory care also refers to services that are provided in a multitude of settings. In addition to traditional hospital-based clinics and programs, ambulatory care is delivered in the home, in private physicians' offices, in prehospital emergency medical services systems, and in community health clinics and freestanding facilities. Of these settings, the majority of ambulatory care is provided in hospital-based programs and private physicians' offices.

Hospital-Based Services

Currently, 4,632, or 73.6 percent, of the 6,291 hospitals have organized outpatient departments; 5,266, or 83.7 percent, of hospitals provide ambulatory surgical services; and 5,197, or 82.6 percent, of hospitals have emergency departments.[2] Since the implementation of the Tax Equity and Fiscal Responsibility Act in 1983 and the prospective payment system that promoted a competitive health care environment, ambulatory care services have witnessed unprecedented growth. As shown in table 2-1, hospital-sponsored and -associated ambulatory care facilities provided 336.2 million services (physician visits, outpatient/ancillary services, and emergency department services) in 1988. This is an increase of 23 percent from 273.2 million services provided in 1983. The numbers and types of ambulatory care programs and services have also increased substantially (table 2-1) since 1983. Most notably, health promotion services and home care programs have increased by 98 percent and 110 percent, respectively.

As indicated previously, enhanced expansion of ambulatory care programs and services has resulted in a notable shifting of patient revenues from once predominantly inpatient services to increasing revenues for hospital-based ambulatory services. Revenues for ambulatory care services from all sources for short-term community hospitals were $37.2 billion in 1988, up from $11.7 billion in 1983.[3] This represents an increase of $25.5 billion and is now equivalent to $126 per service, where service is defined to include the spectrum of visits and ancillary services. Although outpatient revenues are small in comparison to total revenues, they are quite large numerically.

Table 2-1. Hospital-Sponsored Ambulatory Care Utilization Trends, 1983–1988

Visits[a] (in thousands)	1983	1984	1985	1986	1987	1988	Percentage Change 1983-1988
Ambulatory surgery[b]	4,987	5,827	7,308	8,705	9,757	10,589	112.3
Emergency department	77,522	78,492	80,079	82,117	83,478	86,641	11.8
Total outpatient visits[c]	273,168	276,566	282,139	294,633	310,707	336,207	23.1
Outpatient visits[d]	195,646	198,074	202,060	212,516	227,229	249,566	27.5

Programs[e]	1983	1984	1985	1986	1987	1988	Percentage Change 1983-1988
Ambulatory surgery[f]	5,012	5,109	5,245	5,243	5,562	5,266	5.1
Emergency department	5,406	5,397	5,382	5,340	5,572	5,197	(3.9)
Organized outpatient department	3,021	3,191	3,434	3,989	4,242	4,632	53.3
Other outpatient:							
Health promotion	2,559	2,943	3,253	4,424	4,656	5,056	97.6
Home care	920	1,296	1,714	1,986	1,983	1,932	110.0
Hospice	548	616	727	827	820	815	48.7
Rehabilitation	2,146	2,248	2,398	2,329	2,443	2,707	26.1
Psychiatry	1,259	1,292	1,339	1,387	1,428	1,501	19.2
Chemical dependency	1,073	1,134	1,244	1,342	1,416	1,450	35.1

Source: Division of Ambulatory Care, American Hospital Association, 1990.

[a]American Hospital Association's annual survey.

[b]Surgical services provided to patients who do not remain in the hospital overnight.

[c]Visits by patients who are not lodged in the hospital while receiving medical, dental, or other services. Each appearance by an outpatient to each unit of the hospital counts as one outpatient visit.

[d]Refers to outpatient therapy and treatment visits, ancillary service visits, and all other forms of outpatient care not previously defined; also includes ambulatory surgery visits.

[e]American Hospital Association's Hospital Statistics; the number of hospitals reporting for each year was approximately 90 percent.

[f]Information not reported until 1983.

Freestanding Ambulatory Care Facilities

As hospitals have expanded their provision of ambulatory care services, complex and challenging environmental forces have led to widespread entrepreneurial activities in this area. Virtually all ambulatory care activities have now evolved into freestanding settings. Today, these freestanding alternatives have further challenged hospitals to provide ambulatory care services in cost-effective and efficient modes of operation. Although freestanding facilities command a small portion of utilization and revenues relative to hospitals, they have earned a significant and growing place in the health care marketplace. Freestanding facilities that provide urgent, episodic, and primary medical care, commonly referred to as convenience clinics, have increased from fewer than 300 facilities in 1980 to over 3,000 facilities in 1988, an increase of 900 percent.[4] Furthermore, it is estimated that 5,500 such facilities were operational by 1990. In 1980, convenience clinics provided fewer than 5 million patient visits compared to over 43 million visits in 1988. On the basis of year-to-year growth rates, patient visits to convenience clinics were estimated at 63 million by 1990.[5]

Freestanding facilities that provide ambulatory surgery, or surgicenters, have also proliferated. It is estimated that in 1988, over 800 facilities performed in excess of 1.5 million surgical procedures. In 1980, approximately 100 freestanding ambulatory surgery centers were operational; it is predicted that by 1990 approximately 1,200 such facilities will perform nearly 3 million surgical procedures (figure 2-1).[6]

Finally, newer freestanding prototypes have been introduced for ambulatory care programs and services such as diagnostic imaging

Figure 2-1. Hospital-Based and Freestanding Ambulatory Care Providers, 1970–1990

	1970	1980	Est. 1990
I. Hospital-based ambulatory care			
Total facilities	5,859	5,904	5,600
II. Freestanding ambulatory care			
Total providers	7,892	19,516	32,550
1. Freestanding ambulatory surgery centers	1	100	1,200
2. Freestanding ambulatory care centers	N/A	180	5,500
3. Diagnostic imaging centers	N/A	25	6,700
4. Industrial medicine clinics	N/A	5,000	8,000
5. Freestanding cancer centers	N/A	25	200
6. Mobile diagnostic units	N/A	50	750
7. Home care	N/A	2,924	5,800
8. Hospice	N/A	450	1,000
9. Physician group practice	7,891	10,762	15,000

Source: Division of Ambulatory Care and Health Promotion, American Hospital Association, 1989.

centers (figure 2-2). These centers are the products of a combination of forces that have transformed traditional radiology from an inpatient service based on conventional X rays to a multimodal, technology-intensive service offered in a variety of settings. Currently, more than 20 percent of imaging procedures are now performed in freestanding settings, private radiology practices, and diagnostic imaging centers. As technology continues to advance and payers increasingly seek more alternatives at controlling cost escalation, other types of freestanding facilities will emerge as well.

Physician Practices

Solo and group practices have long established themselves as the predominant deliverers of ambulatory care services. However, these entities are now experiencing the dramatic restructuring affecting other ambulatory care providers. Growth in the number of physicians is greater than population growth, physician practice affiliations are shifting as a result of increased competition, and cost-containment pressures are leading to more restrictive reimbursement policies. Currently, the practice of solo medicine is in decline while physician group practices are experiencing phenomenal growth.

Group practices are emerging as increasingly powerful entities because larger patient volumes substantiate the demand for acquiring technologies once considered the domain of hospital-based ambulatory care programs. Generally, a group practice consists of three or more physicians who share the patient care and business aspects of a medical practice. The American Medical Association indicated that in 1987 physician group practices numbered 17,556—an increase of 61.3 percent since 1980.[7] Hospitals have shown more interest in affiliating with or developing group practices in order to maintain and perhaps even increase

Figure 2-2. Ambulatory Care Facility Development, 1987–1988

	1987	1988	Percentage Change
I. Ambulatory care centers			
Completed	143	141	(1.4)
Under development	235	281	19.6
II. Diagnostic imaging centers			
Completed	107	180	68.2
Under development	164	230	40.2
III. Medical office buildings			
Completed	152	188	23.7
Under development	249	291	16.9

Source: Adapted from *Modern Healthcare* Construction and Architects Survey, 1989 and 1988.

market share. Hospitals have acknowledged widespread acquisition of group practices and have entered into formalized joint-venture relationships to ensure captivity of such markets.

Evidence of the powerful organization of group practices is apparent by numerous large groups that have expanded to include not only traditional clinic-type operations, but ambulatory surgery capabilities; diagnostic imaging services; urgent care programs; physical therapy, outpatient rehabilitation and sports medicine services; and cardiovascular diagnostic services. Because these groups are often the initial entrance point for a number of patients, group practices can offer ease and convenience for patients that hospitals and other freestanding providers are seeking to attract. With the increasing movement toward multispecialty group practices, their survival will depend in part on their efforts to successfully deliver comprehensive, state-of-the-art services to ambulatory care patients.

A Micro Perspective: Specific Programs and Services

The previous broad overview of the ambulatory care marketplace reflects the tremendous growth and diversity of ambulatory settings. Even though ambulatory care now includes newer, more specialized areas such as outpatient cardiovascular testing, industrial/occupational medicine, pain management, and behavioral medicine, the traditional forms of ambulatory care still comprise the bulk of patient visits and testing. Ambulatory surgery, emergency services, laboratory and radiology services, for instance, typically comprise over 70 percent of a hospital's outpatient utilization. These areas, however, are undergoing tremendous change and will create unique challenges for automating information gathering and reporting.

Ambulatory Surgery

Of all ambulatory services offered today, ambulatory surgery can be described as experiencing the greatest growth as well as undergoing the most profound changes. Preferred by an increasing number of third-party payers, physicians, and patients, ambulatory surgery eliminates the cost of an overnight stay and offers convenience to both physicians and patients.

The trend toward increased utilization of ambulatory surgery procedures persists for all hospital types, including not-for-profit and investor-owned hospitals. In 1988, 47 percent of these procedures, or 10.6 million, were performed on an outpatient basis. By comparison, only 16 percent of these procedures, or 3.2 million, were performed in 1980—an increase of 231 percent.[8] Among hospital bed-size groupings, all hospitals are performing in excess of 40 percent outpatient procedures. In various regions of the country, it has been reported that some hospitals are already reaching a 60 percent level of outpatient surgical procedures, which is predicted as the industry average by 1995.

The proliferation of freestanding surgical centers, estimated at over 800 in 1988, has caused an obvious erosion of some patients from traditional hospital-based programs. Although freestanding surgical centers performed in excess of 1.5 million procedures in 1988, hospitals still hold more than an 80 percent share of the surgical procedure marketplace.[9]

Continued development of new technologies and expanded payment initiatives for ambulatory surgery, including increased provider (physician) acceptance, will no doubt shift the majority of previous inpatient caseloads to outpatient settings. The number of surgical procedures that can be appropriately conducted in outpatient environments, often the subject of great debate, exceeds several hundred in number.

Technological enhancements notwithstanding, perhaps the greatest movement toward outpatient surgery for hospitals will result from the enactment of the Omnibus Budget Reconciliation Act (OBRA) of 1986. This measure calls for the development of a prospective payment system for reimbursing all Medicare outpatient services and, until fully implemented, sets forth new regulations by which hospitals will be reimbursed for providing ambulatory surgical services to Medicare beneficiaries.

Several key features of these new regulations will force hospitals to implement operational changes to accommodate requirements for medical records, billing information systems, and other areas to ensure payment.

One important feature of OBRA is that outpatient procedures must be coded according to the Health Care Financing Administration's Common Procedural Coding System for Ambulatory Surgery Procedures (HCPCS). All procedures must be coded, whether or not the procedure is approved by the Ambulatory Surgery Center (ASC). Hospitals will be required to continue submitting ICD-9-CM diagnosis codes; however, ICD-9 procedural codes are no longer required. The Health Care Financing Administration has stated that it will use an Outpatient Code Editor that will edit the UB-82 form and will reject those claims that are miscoded. To this end, providers will have to develop management information systems that provide a "crosswalk" between coding systems, as well as conversion tables to expedite the interface between coding systems.

Emergency Department Services

Emergency departments provide a mix of services for both emergent patients and patients requiring primary medical care. Despite the emergency department's role in providing care to great numbers of out-patients, many institutions recognize the emergency department as an inpatient service. This is because the emergency department is the single largest source of inpatient admissions.[10] Currently, 40 percent of total hospital admissions nationwide are generated from the emergency department. Similarly, 10 to 20 percent of emergency department visits result in an inpatient admission. Although emergency departments represent nearly 30 percent of total ambulatory care utilization in hospitals, emergency departments account for significant volumes of other diagnostic/ancillary utilization. It is estimated that as much as 70 percent of outpatient radiology procedures and as much as 40 percent of outpatient laboratory procedures are generated by emergency department patients.[11]

Despite the success that emergency departments have enjoyed, their future will be confronted with many challenges. Today, there is growing concern among many third-party payers that emergency departments are inappropriately utilized, causing unneeded and expensive expenditures. Critics contend that as many as 70 percent of current emergency department patients could be treated in more appropriate, cost-effective settings. Various payers are now implementing more stringent requirements as to what constitutes an appropriate versus an inappropriate patient visit, and they are denying payment for certain types of services. In addition, a number of health maintenance organization and preferred provider organization plans now discourage emergency department use and have begun to institute deductibles for patients who are inappropriately referred for emergency department care.

As these cost-containment strategies become widespread, national emergency department utilization will stabilize and then begin to decline. It is projected that emergency department visits will stabilize in the early 1990s and then decrease for several years. This trend will in turn have a negative financial impact on hospitals. The American Hospital Association estimates that the emergency department contributes 3 to 7 percent of revenues indirectly through ancillaries, patient days, and supplies.[12] To survive in this environment in the future, hospitals will have to ensure that their emergency departments are oriented toward a strong consumer approach; pricing of services must be based on the actual cost of providing such care; and some services that do not achieve profitability may have to be eliminated or merged with other facilities.

Radiology and Related Services

Radiologic diagnostic and imaging capabilities have emerged as one of the most exciting and challenging areas in hospital outpatient expansion during the past five years. Radiology has been transformed from a level of routine, simple diagnostic technology to one that is extremely high-technology based. The shift of traditional diagnostic examinations to digital modalities such as magnetic resonance imaging (MRI), computerized tomography (CT), and ultrasound will forever change the landscape of radiological technology. Advances in development of multimodal techniques will greatly affect the treatment regimens of patients, moving radiology into the forefront as one of the first tools to be incorporated in the diagnosis and management of patients. The emergence of positron emission tomography (PET) imaging, which provides three-dimensional metabolic and functional views of organs, and lithotripsy, which uses "shock wave" ultrasound to destruct kidney stones and gallstones, are but two examples.

The provision of radiology and diagnostic imaging services is further challenged by the manner in which these services can be provided. In addition to hospital-based radiology departments, services are increasingly being developed in freestanding imaging centers and on the road via mobile vans. For hospitals, this situation is a difficult one; radiology departments often suffer financial losses because of their high overhead associated with staffing of personnel and technology costs. As lower-cost, high-volume procedures are provided outside of the hospital, higher costs per procedure are incurred, which increases the level of operating losses.

In the future, hospitals must brace for reimbursement changes in the outpatient radiology area. Already, diagnostic imaging centers have witnessed 5 to 10 percent declines in reimbursement due to changes in payment regulations.[13] Several strategies can be employed to assist in operational decision making. These should include performing cost accounting of services to more precisely define departmental productivity; conducting profit and loss analyses for each imaging modality to determine if certain cost controls should be employed; considering new alternatives to acquire technology or increase departmental profitability, such as equipment leasing, contract management and joint ventures; and reviewing local and regionalized service offerings, such as multi-institutional development of MRI services (which may be the only alternative for some to achieve profitable operations).

Laboratory Services

Clinical laboratory testing, provided in hospitals and physicians' offices and by independent laboratories, is one segment of the ambulatory care spectrum undergoing rapid change on a daily basis. It is a fiercely competitive marketplace, characterized by an endless number of providers in a matured environment.

Even though the clinical laboratory testing market is an enormous industry, the exact number of tests performed by the various testing entities is unknown. It is estimated, however, that the market is approximately $20 billion annually, with the biggest share—$13 billion—provided by hospitals.[14] Approximately 6 million tests are performed annually; roughly 50 to 57 percent of tests are performed in hospitals, 25 to 30 percent are performed in independent laboratories, and the remaining 15 to 20 percent are conducted in physicians' offices. According to the most recent estimates, 74 percent of all clinical laboratories in the United States have witnessed increasing volumes in tests conducted since 1984–1986. It is predicted that hospital laboratory testing will increase at an annual rate of 5 percent, whereas physicians' offices and group practices will experience annual growth of 16 and 19 percent, respectively.[15]

The growth of total laboratory testing over the past three decades has consistently been measured in double-digit figures. Although growth will continue in the future, massive restructuring and consolidation among the various players will proliferate. For hospitals, ongoing changes in payment systems are transforming laboratories from profit-generating centers to cost centers. Prior to the implementation of the prospective payment system, hospital laboratories generated approximately 12 percent of total hospital revenue; laboratories now cost money instead of generating it.

Overall, the number of hospital and independent laboratories has decreased over 30 percent in the past decade as a result of consolidations, acquisitions, and joint ventures between competitors. These changes have come about because profits are directly related to economies of scale; most tests provide slim profit margins and are dependent on tremendous amounts of volume to sustain a program's viability. Conversely, the number of physicians'-office laboratories has increased dramatically, as has the range of testing available within these offices. This growth has occurred because of patients' and physicians' desires for quicker turnaround of tests, enhanced medical technology that has made office testing easier, and a somewhat favorable reimbursement climate that has helped boost the profitability of such laboratories.

In the future, cost pressures and reimbursement challenges will continue to threaten the operational effectiveness of hospital laboratory testing. More tests will be provided on a decentralized basis because of the advances of simple instrumentation and test kits that can be performed by patients at home. To remain an active player in the field, hospitals will have to implement a number of innovative strategies. First, productivity and efficiency gains will be targeted through cost reduction efforts; independent laboratories will be used for certain types of testing and contract management will be employed to assume the costs of overall administration and training programs. Equipment upgrading and computerization of testing and results reporting may also be viable options. Finally, a structure may be created that enables the hospital to act as a reference laboratory for physicians and industry.

Ambulatory Care Challenges

Challenges associated with ambulatory care growth from both macro and micro perspectives portray a scenario of success for many hospitals and providers. Yet, concurrent with this growth are many diverse and complex challenges that must be confronted. These challenges include the impending reform of Medicare Part B reimbursement, cost-containment initiatives by other third parties, productivity assessment and enhancement, and quality of care validation, as well as responding to an increasingly changing patient mix. Thus, developing and managing the necessary information capabilities to care for ambulatory patients will be imperative to survive in this environment of profound change.

Medicare Outpatient Reform

Among the health care services covered by Medicare, reimbursement for hospital outpatient services has shown the highest rate of growth since the program's inception. With the advent of the prospective payment system, hospital outpatient expenditures have increased phenomenally. In 1988, Medicare charges for hospital outpatient services amounted to $7 billion—an increase of 112 percent from $3.3 billion in 1983.[16]

The prospective payment system has created incentives for hospitals to hold down costs, because they earn a profit when their costs fall below the prospective payment or absorb a loss when their costs exceed the payment threshold. As a result, providers have been shortening lengths of stay, reducing ancillary services, and fostering outpatient alternatives for care. According to an interim report on the impact of prospective payment on hospitals, a number of preliminary findings indicate reasons why ambulatory care is one of the fastest-growing segments of the health care industry:

1. There are direct financial incentives for hospitals to shift care to ambulatory settings when it is clinically appropriate and cost-efficient.
2. Surgical and diagnostic innovations have enabled hospitals to perform more procedures on an ambulatory basis.
3. Utilization review policies have influenced the Medicare patient mix in hospitals since preadmission review now encourages treatment in the most appropriate and cost-effective setting.
4. The addition of ambulatory surgical benefits and the repeal of the deductible for home health services have encouraged greater outpatient use.[17]

As discussed earlier, the Health Care Financing Administration has long recognized the need to create further incentives for efficiency and productivity; it appears that the early 1990s will be the beginning of payment reform for all ambulatory care services. (See chapter 8 for a full discussion of prospective payment.)

Cost-Containment Initiatives

It is estimated that in excess of $5 billion is spent each year for health care services. If today's annual rate of health care spending continues at the current rate of 7 to 10 percent, it is predicted that health care will represent approximately 28 percent of the gross national product by the early part of the 21st century.[18] Although numerous reasons abound for the explosive growth in health care costs, widespread attention is now being focused on every effort to contain these expenditures.

Currently, two-thirds of the health care provided in the United States is funded by employers via insurance benefits to employees. In order to stem the increases in costs, many employers are offering their employees incentives for using services that substitute for inpatient services. In some cases, they are demanding that outpatient alternatives be used exclusively. Because employers represent one of the most significant buyers in the marketplace, their influence in determining what services will be utilized is quite significant. They are becoming increasingly sophisticated in purchasing health care services and evaluating services received.

Although companies provide coverage for outpatient alternatives, most companies continue to reimburse employees for these services at the same rate as inpatient care. This trend alone is mainly responsible for the claim that outpatient care, while appropriate, is not a less costly alternative to inpatient services. Companies are, however, attempting to ensure that expenditures are warranted. Over 90 percent of companies now require mandatory second opinions for surgical care or offer financial incentives for employees who obtain second opinions on their own behalf.[19]

In addition to certain changes in health benefit design plans, a number of companies now require mandatory cost sharing from employees who utilize certain types of health care services. Most companies require employees to pay 20 percent of charges for most services subject to a copayment. Copayments, premiums, and deductibles are also common forms of employee cost sharing that are being utilized more frequently and at increasing rates by employers.

In recent years, industry has embraced the concept that in order to reduce health care expenditures, utilization of services must be controlled. Thus "managed care" has evolved, and many companies, insurers, and payers have implemented various managed care protocols. In terms of providing ambulatory care services, preservice certification requirements will allow payers to question elective ambulatory services and identify patients whose condition could be unusually expensive, more expensive than anticipated, or require a greater intensity of follow-up.

Productivity Assessment

The assessment and management of productivity in the ambulatory care setting will be a difficult challenge for hospitals in the 1990s. Because ambulatory care is provided to numerous patients and often consists of multiple procedures performed in various departments or settings, it is highly labor-intensive. In addition, because ambulatory services have low margins per unit of service, it is difficult to maintain overall program viability; the level of services performed often exceeds the level of available resources.

To achieve the critical balance between improved productivity and the attainment of high-quality patient care in the ambulatory setting, hospitals will have to adopt a number of innovative strategies. First, hospital executive management will have to embrace a broad set of goals and policies for ambulatory care delivery. This measure will determine to a greater extent the efficiency and effectiveness with which each institution can organize resources to deliver and manage ambulatory care patients. Second, productivity management programs will need to be implemented to ensure that various services are delivered to ambulatory patients on a clinically justified basis, in addition to being delivered in the most appropriate and cost-effective manner. Finally, operational efficiency must be achieved through high-level managerial development. To achieve such operational productivity, the development of support systems that allow employees to attain their full working potential must be initiated.

Because productivity standards are now viewed as critical variables in the delivery of ambulatory care, adherence to these measures will determine the ultimate success of each ambulatory program or service. Once ambulatory growth stabilizes and revenue maximization is achieved, the only viable option to improve operational effectiveness will be cost reduction through productivity improvement.

Defining Quality of Service

Despite the constant debate as to what variables constitute an accurate definition of quality in health care delivery, greater attention to quality issues in the ambulatory setting will be exercised by various providers. This represents a formidable task, because systematic review of outpatients is difficult to achieve. For instance, the large volume of patients treated in ambulatory settings does not lend itself to total review of all patients; treatment outcomes may be difficult to ascertain; medical record charting is often incomplete and noncomputerized; and charting is often very subjective in terms of factors contributing to a patient's outcome.

Because quality of patient care is subjective as well as objective in nature, a definition of quality in ambulatory care delivery will no doubt include all of these parameters. The Quality Assurance Committee of the Society for Ambulatory Care Professionals, a personal membership organization of the American Hospital Association, contends that quality in the ambulatory care setting equals attributes associated with that care. Thus, attributes of high-quality health care can be measured in such a way as to demonstrate the positive level of quality or, conversely, the lack of quality. Each attribute is one that a reasonable purchaser of health care associates with good quality and expects to have provided. To this end, attributes include the effectiveness of care delivered or technical competency; service or the acceptability of services; access or the availability of services; consideration of the value-added concept; and continuity of care.[20]

The movement toward defining and measuring quality will also create challenges for hospitals regarding quality's relationship to profits. Increasingly, some payers are contemplating a philosophy that high-quality care costs much less in the long term than lower-quality care. In other words, high-quality care reduces the costs of low-quality care, for example, less cost for inspection, maintenance, and replacement of technology; and a higher-quality product or service may increase the likelihood of charging a higher price for a valued service. Thus, a higher quality of services can actually cost less and generate higher profits. Particularly in the ambulatory care arena, where services are more price-sensitive than in the inpatient setting, hospitals must continually enhance their quality of care assessments if they wish to remain a strong competitor in the marketplace.

Changing Patient Mix

A number of forces are currently challenging the health care industry's ability to meet the demands of specific population segments. The tremendous increase in the number of AIDS patients, the increased prevalence of disease among the aged, homelessness, and the uninsured and underinsured populations pose serious problems for providers. Ambulatory care settings will be most affected, because the initial and sometimes only points of entry into the health care system for these patients are the emergency department and community health centers. For instance, home care programs are actively being used for the treatment location of choice for patients with AIDS and for the chronically ill. As these patients multiply in number and the population ages, the service capacity necessary to care for all patients will be strained and the profitability of overall operations will be questionable for some institutions.

The fundamental inpatient to outpatient shift is also creating a new category of ambulatory patients not seen five years ago. Generally, these patients have very complex medical problems and may be dependent on sophisticated technological equipment each day. While undergoing ambulatory procedures or testing, they require more preparation time, transportation time, and increased supervision by nursing and technical personnel. Thus, the mix of these patients in ambulatory settings will create challenges in achieving productivity standards and operational efficiency targets.

The Management of Information

The environmental factors influencing the rate of ambulatory care growth will mandate the development of information systems for ambulatory care settings. Unfortunately, many of the current systems are predominantly manual because the investment in ambulatory information systems has lagged behind that of inpatient information systems. This alone has caused severe shortcomings in the ability of each facility to adequately manage the tremendous amounts of ambulatory care data. [To this end, many institutions will realize that a fully integrated management information system (MIS) will ultimately be required. A fully integrated MIS will combine clinical, financial, and operational data for day-to-day management issues and strategic planning purposes.]

Conclusion

Ambulatory care, which is becoming the key point of health care delivery, will continue to expand and to offer numerous challenges in terms of information services requirements. Whether care is provided in freestanding facilities or, like most ambulatory care services, in hospital-based programs or private physicians' offices, cost-effective and efficient delivery of services will be essential.

References

1. Meshenberg, K. A., and Burns, L. *Hospital Ambulatory Care: Making it Work.* Chicago: American Hospital Publishing, 1984.

2. American Hospital Association. *Hospital Statistics, 1989, 1988, and 1983.* Chicago: AHA, 1989, 1988, and 1984.

3. American Hospital Association. *National Hospital Panel Survey, 1988 and 1984.* Chicago: AHA, 1988 and 1984.

4. SMG Marketing Group. *Freestanding Ambulatory Care Center Report.* Chicago: SMG, 1987.

5. *Freestanding Ambulatory Care Center Report.*

6. SMG Marketing Group. *Freestanding Outpatient Surgery Center Report*. Chicago: SMG, 1987.

7. American Medical Association. *The Environment of Medicine, 1985*. Chicago: AMA, 1985.

8. American Hospital Association. *Hospital Statistics, 1989 and 1981*. Chicago: AHA, 1989 and 1981.

9. Ambulatory care growth continues. *Outreach* 10(1):2, Jan.–Feb. 1989.

10. Matson, T. A. *The Hospital Emergency Department: Returning to Financial Viability*. Chicago: American Hospital Publishing, 1986.

11. Matson, T. A. Rethinking the delivery of ambulatory care: hospital-based versus freestanding alternatives. Presentation, "Penetrating the Alternate Site Marketplace Conference," Biomedical Business International, San Francisco, Sept. 15, 1987.

12. Matson, Rethinking the delivery of ambulatory care.

13. Sabatino, F. Survey: managed care led '89 diversification improvements. *Hospitals* 64(1):58, Jan. 5, 1990.

14. Biomedical Business International. Clinical laboratory services industry. BBI report no. 7076. Tustin, CA: BBI, 1987.

15. Biomedical Business International, report no. 7076.

16. Health Care Financing Administration, Office of the Actuary.

17. American Hospital Association Division of Ambulatory Care. *Home Care Survey*. Chicago: AHA, 1986.

18. National health expenditures 1986. *Health Care Financing Review* 1986. [No further information available.]

19. The Business Roundtable Health, Welfare, and Retirement Income Task Force Report: Corporate Health-Care-Cost Management and Private Sector Initiatives. Indianapolis: The Business Roundtable, 1987.

20. Quality Assurance Committee, Society for Ambulatory Care Professionals, American Hospital Association, Chicago, 1988.

Chapter 3

Ambulatory Care Information Systems

Helen L. Hill and Gerald R. Mathys

Fueled by competition and by the need to contain costs and conserve other scarce resources, the demand for more and better health care information systems and services continues to rise. On the other hand, after 20 years of exposure to information systems, hospitals, clinics, physicians' offices, and health care insurers still have largely manual operations. (Health care insurers include health maintenance organizations [HMOs], preferred provider organizations [PPOs], and individual practice arrangements [IPAs].) They have not invested heavily in automation and have not fully understood or used the products they have bought.

Health care institutions, in particular those in ambulatory care, need to learn to use automation more effectively, starting with basic operational support of financial, administrative, and clinical areas, through use of information as a management tool and as a strategic resource. Until they have learned to do this effectively, even the best products will give poor results.

This chapter will examine ambulatory care information systems as an element of the health care information systems market. It will discuss the state of the art in health care and ambulatory care information systems; examine recent technological developments and their probable impacts; and then focus on future opportunities and trends in these markets.

Problems and Opportunities

Five years ago, in an article on future directions for ambulatory care information systems, Donald M. Steinwachs wrote that ambulatory care organizations had been reluctant to invest in management information systems (MIS), due to concerns about cost and about the ability of MIS to support critical management decision making in areas other than finance. He predicted that exciting areas for growth would include:

- Integration of clinical and management systems
- Increased use of decision support systems
- New technologies for networking systems

He urged that computer-based methodologies for examining the effectiveness of ambulatory care practices be developed. These were to be based on potential cost impacts or on improvements in quality of care.[1]

Some work has been done in these areas, but principally on the in-patient side of the business, where regulatory and competitive pressures have been greatest, and even there, no widely accepted methods have been routinely included in commercially available software.

The ambulatory care information systems on the market today are often narrow in scope. The systems of the future must be broad in scope and rich in function. They must address more of the unique needs of this market.

The Unique Needs of Ambulatory Care Information Systems

The information systems serving the ambulatory care market fall into the same broad categories as the traditional hospital information system (HIS): financial, clinical, and administrative applications. However, significant differences between the acute care and ambulatory care environments have created the need for highly specialized ambulatory care information systems. These differences include the structures and purposes of the organizations served; federal, state, and third-party regulatory requirements; and the patient care environment itself. Ambulatory care often involves numerous episodes of care by widely scattered providers over long periods of time. Acute care does not.

Traditional hospital information systems do not meet these unique needs. For example, inpatient billing systems do not post cash at the procedure level. Outpatient services often require HCPCS codes instead of ICD-9-CM codes as billing documentation. Few acute care systems can accommodate the complex pricing and reporting needs of the mul-tientity, multilocation organizations prevalent in ambulatory care. Still fewer can generate profit and loss statements for the individual physi-cian within a group of specialists within a multispecialty clinic. Practice management systems and HMO enrollment systems are not general HIS offerings. Few automated systems supporting HMOs and PPOs can accommodate multiple practice models or multiple plans. Clinical encounters are usually documented within systems by admission or by individual visit, not by ambulatory patient groups or by program (for example, oncology) over extended time periods.

Investing in Health Care Information Systems

Before moving on to specific information systems for ambulatory care, it is helpful to consider the broader health care environment and its experience with information systems. Historically, the health care industry has not used computers to their full potential. Health care lags behind other industries in investments in automation. Studies show that the hospital segment, the largest user of automation in the health care industry, has invested less than 2 percent of its total operating budget in automation, whereas manufacturing and banking have invested more than twice that rate.[2] One long-term consequence of this low level of investment has been that even the most sophisticated hospital administrators and managers have comparatively little experience in evaluating, implementing, and effectively managing computer systems.

With the institution of prospective reimbursement in 1983, this situation began to improve. Hospitals began to invest significantly greater percentages of their operating budgets in automation; these budgets rose from 1.9 percent in 1982 to 2.5 percent ($3.6 billion) in 1987. An additional $1 billion in capital was spent in 1987 to support information systems efforts, bringing the 1987 total spent on automation to $4.8 billion.[3]

Although the largest single component of hospital computer expenditures continues to be in the area of patient accounting, other clinical applications such as patient care, laboratory, and pharmacy systems have grown substantially in recent years.

At the end of 1988, 95.8 percent of the nation's 5,611 community hospitals had computerized patient accounting applications; 35.1 percent had automated patient care systems; 44.8 percent had automated pharmacy systems; and 32.4 percent had automated laboratory systems.[4] Data in table 3-1 show the relationship between hospital size and extent of automation in major application areas.

Growth Projections

The number of hospitals automating patient care functions and pharmacy and laboratory services is expected to increase more than 80 percent by 1993. By 1993, about half of all patient accounting users will also have computerized patient care and laboratory systems, compared with less than one-third in 1986. Nearly 75 percent of patient accounting users in 1993 will have automated pharmacy systems, compared with 38.8 percent in 1988. Because patient accounting is already automated in 95.8

Table 3-1. Community Hospital Computer Users in 1988, by Application and Bed Size

Bed Size	All Community Hospitals	Patient Accounting		Patient Care		Laboratory		Pharmacy		Admitting	
		Number	% of All	Number	% of All	Number	% of All	Number	% of All	Number	% of All
Under 100	2,574	2,350	91.3%	225	8.7%	225	8.7%	550	21.4%	1,825	70.9%
100–199	1,352	1,344	99.4%	510	37.7%	415	30.7%	668	49.4%	1,151	85.1%
200–299	746	746	100.0%	500	67.0%	418	56.0%	537	72.0%	701	94.0%
300–399	432	432	100.0%	345	79.9%	332	76.9%	343	79.4%	424	98.1%
400–499	207	270	100.0%	169	81.6%	167	80.7%	174	84.1%	204	98.6%
500 & over	300	299	99.7%	223	74.3%	263	87.7%	243	81.0%	288	96.0%
Total	5,611	5,378	95.8%	1,972	35.1%	1,820	32.4%	2,515	44.8%	4,593	81.9%

Source: Copyright ©1989 by Sheldon I. Dorenfest & Associates, Ltd. Reprinted with permission.

percent of all community hospitals, this application area will grow more slowly than applications that are less widely used.[5]

The health care market for computer-related products and services is rapidly growing. One of the fastest-growing segments is expenditures for turnkey systems, a major subset of the "Software and Management Services" category shown in table 3-2, which shows market share trends among major categories of computer products and services.

Software companies have recognized the potential of this relatively untapped market and are now developing more products for the hospital segment. Forecasts for 1993 project health care expenditures for computer-related products and services to reach $6 billion. In contrast, 1988 expenditures were $3.7 billion, including ambulatory care.[6] Data in figure 3-1 show the projected distribution of these funds in 1993, with expected growth over 1988 levels. Hospitals' expenditures for ambulatory care information systems are included in the "Other Applications and Consulting" category.

Overall Industry Needs

Today, health care providers are prepared to spend more on automation, but only if better products become available. The limitation is not money but the quality of available software. New products must be created to meet the challenges of the 1990s. Industry needs include:

- Multientity, multilocation, multiuser capabilities
- Integrated access to centralized patient information (clinical, administrative, and financial)
- Timely access to patient treatment data
- Extensive clinical and administrative applications
- Automated techniques for information management and analysis
- Methods for review of health care resource utilization by physicians, managed care plan members, employees, and specific market segments
- Common definitions of such units of measure as ambulatory patient groups, encounters, and intensity of service
- Productivity measurement systems
- Modular, flexible, user-modifiable systems to accommodate future change

Systems Deficiencies

Products on the market fall far short of health care organizations' needs. Deficiencies in these systems include:

- Lack of comprehensive functionality and expandability
- Past failures (vendors have oversold systems; products have failed)

Table 3-2. Health Care Computing Market by Product Type ($ in millions)

Product Type	1980 Sales	1980 Share of Market	1985 Sales	1985 Share of Market	1986 Sales	1986 Share of Market	1987 Sales	1987 Share of Market	1988 Sales	1988 Share of Market
Computer hardware sold direct	$ 535.0	49.1%	$1,200.0	42.1%	$1,250.0	39.1%	$1,300.0	36.6%	$1,375.0	36.9%
Shared computer services	290.0	26.6%	400.0	14.0%	350.0	10.9%	275.0	7.8%	225.0	6.0%
Software and management services	225.0	20.6%	1,115.0	39.1%	1,425.0	44.5%	1,775.0	50.0%	1,900.0	51.1%
Consulting	40.0	3.7%	135.0	4.8%	175.0	5.5%	200.0	5.6%	225.0	6.0%
Total hospital sales	$1,090.0	100.0%	$2,850.0	100.0%	$3,200.0	100.0%	$3,550.0	100.0%	$3,725.0	100.0%
Computer hardware sold through value added retailers	$ 140.0	12.8%	$385.0	13.5%	$475.0	14.8%	$600.0	16.9%	$700.0	18.8%

Source: Copyright ©1989 by Sheldon I. Dorenfest & Associates, Ltd. Reprinted with permission.

Figure 3-1. 1993 Expenditures by Application

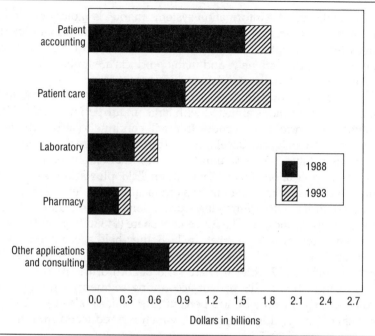

Source: Copyright ©1989 by Sheldon I. Dorenfest & Associates, Ltd. Reprinted with permission.

- Inability of purchasers to differentiate among products
- Lack of truly integrated products
- Incompatible hardware and software in the complex multivendor environment common today
- High cost
- Inability to realize benefits

Current Ambulatory Care Information Systems

Today, over 1,000 vendors offer software products and services to the ambulatory care market. Some of these vendors offer only one or two applications to highly specialized segments of the market. Very few of these vendors offer a comprehensive range of products. Few of these vendors have revenues of over $10 million, few are successful, and few have a national focus.

The most frequently offered applications are group practice billing (200), appointment scheduling (180), and HMO enrollment and claims processing (140). Besides hospital information systems, different vendors and products serve the solo and small group practices, the medium-sized group practices, and the large, multispecialty groups/clinics.

Growth Projections

The ambulatory care information systems market is rapidly expanding, and it is still in an evolutionary stage. Significant additional growth is forecasted. As chapter 9 will describe, market entry requires limited capital; many vendors are new; and many products are limited or specialty-niche systems, usually standalone.

The driving force in the market appears likely to be the 50 to 100 health care institutions affiliated with large, multispecialty clinics. These institutions control the revenues that will continue to attract the attention, and research and development funds, of the major suppliers.

Data in table 3-3 show trends in sales, market share, and growth for major applications from 1979 through 1988, plus a forecast for 1993. Ambulatory care information system acquisitions by hospitals are included under "Other Emerging Applications and Consulting." In 1979, emerging applications held a 5.3 percent share ($48 million) of the health care computer industry market. In 1988, they held a 19.5 percent share ($725 million). By 1993, this segment is projected to grow by 120.7 percent to reach a 26.7 percent share ($1.6 billion) of the market.

In contrast, the HIS patient accounting segment of the market is projected to grow only by 10.3 percent ($1.6 billion), also for a 26.7 percent share during the same period, which is a reduction from the 43.7 percent share of 1987.

Under the assumption that "complete" products (that is, those with both ambulatory care and acute care components) are important to market dominance, at least two ambulatory care vendors, Cycare ($68 million in 1987 revenues) and IDX ($45 million), are now offering acute care HIS products. In addition, three major acute care HIS vendors (SMS, Baxter, and Unisys) are offering physician office systems, physician billing systems, or hospital–physician links. (See chapter 9 for more details on these vendors.) Most health care institutions and most hospital information system suppliers are waiting for the market to develop.

Systems Deficiencies

Ambulatory care systems needs are usually met by standalone systems, by in-house development, or by use of existing patient care or patient accounting systems or vendors. Without major alterations, today's acute care HIS products meet only a few of the special needs of the ambulatory care market. High-priority ambulatory care requirements often have lower priorities in hospital corporations' strategic information systems plans.

In the ambulatory setting, opinion has not settled yet even on the appropriate method of classifying data: by visit/episode of service, by ambulatory visit group, or by some other method. Criteria are needed

Table 3-3. Market Size and Growth by Application ($ in millions)

Application	1979		1986		1987		Estimated 1988			Forecast 1993		
	Sales	Share of Market	Sales	Share of Market	Sales	Share of Market	Sales	Share of Market	Growth over 1987	Sales	Share of Market	Growth over 1988
Patient accounting	$635.0	70.6%	$1,525.0	47.7%	$1,550.0	43.7%	$1,450.0	38.9%	(6.5%)	$1,600.0	26.7%	10.3%
Patient care	147.0	16.3%	725.0	22.6%	850.0	23.9%	925.0	24.8%	8.8%	1,800.0	30.0%	94.6%
Laboratory	55.0	6.1%	285.0	8.9%	350.0	9.9%	425.0	11.4%	21.4%	675.0	11.2%	58.9%
Pharmacy	15.0	1.7%	140.0	4.4%	175.0	4.9%	200.0	5.4%	14.3%	325.0	5.4%	62.5%
Other emerging applications and consulting	48.0	5.3%	525.0	16.4%	625.0	17.6%	725.0	19.5%	16.0%	1,600.0	26.7%	120.7%
Total	$900.0	100.0%	$3,200.0	100.0%	$3,550.0	100.0%	$3,725.0	100.0%	4.9%	$6,000.0	100.0%	61.1%

for linking services into episodes of care; multiple diagnoses must be handled per episode; whether to treat chronic conditions as single events or as a series of events over time needs to be resolved. Case mix measures are needed for capitated populations, and cost models for individual practices need to be determined.

Information system deficiencies include limited pricing and discounting features; inability to handle the complex reimbursement constraints associated with fee-for-service billing, managed care (fee-for-service), managed care (capitation); lack of multientity support; lack of an automated ambulatory care medical record with information on multiple episodes of care; limited and oversold hospital–physician links; limited clinical analysis applications; and poor to nonexistent integration of computer systems, at the hardware, software application, and information levels.

A significant problem with commercial software available to health care today is that very little manual function is actually automated. Also, because integration does not work and interfacing is a poor substitute, redundant data are stored in multiple ancillary systems and the ideal of uniting clinical, financial, and administrative data for a patient in a timely fashion is far from being achieved.

These shortcomings provide many opportunities and challenges for vendors to improve current products.

Hospital–Physician Links

In highly competitive environments, hospitals often identify physicians as primary target markets and develop marketing programs, including computer-based information systems and consulting services, specifically for them. Physicians often get free computers as part of "hospital–physician links."[7] These links strive to provide patient registration, admissions, insurance, and demographic data to the physician's office, and sometimes they allow remote registration/admission from the physician's office. Access to laboratory and radiology results and to electronic mail systems is often available. Less frequently, hospitals offer access to appointment scheduling, billing, and other financial systems.

Benefits to hospitals may include increased referrals, occupancy, and revenues.[8] Addition of one new family practice physician to a hospital staff can be expected to bring in an additional $300,000 per year in direct admission revenues and another $300,000 in referrals to its specialists.[9]

Research by Sheldon I. Dorenfest indicates a heavy and increasing hospital demand for these hospital–physician links. However, user expectations of these links may be unrealistically high. Features and functions provided are often rudimentary: read-only access to limited data; remote printing of summary-level reports or of individual test results, with nothing in between. Statistics and graphic displays of data are rare. Systems provided through these links are not integrated today; they are merely connected electronically. The user with access to five different functions may need to know unique protocols for five separate systems. Adding new applications may not be simple or cheap. Today, extensive and expensive customizations are required to go beyond this point. Complex data ownership, data privacy, access, security, and legal liability issues need to be worked through as well. Until better products are available, hospitals should be careful not to oversell these links to their physicians.

Providing high-quality information and comprehensive computer services to physicians will become increasingly important. Computer use by private physician practices is projected to rise from 36 percent in 1986 to 80 percent in 1990.[10] In addition, computer literacy among physicians is rising. In 1987, 64 percent of all U.S. medical schools offered electives in the use of computers in medicine, up from 34 percent in 1983.[11] As computer use and levels of expertise increase, demands for more sophisticated information services will evolve. Hospitals and vendors should position themselves to provide more extensive, comprehensive, and user-friendly information systems and services. The future is very bright for good products in this area, particularly as more patient data are automated.

Managed Care Information Systems

According to a recent survey conducted by the Washington Business Group on Health, the majority of HMOs are unable to get data from their information systems on group-specific utilization of inpatient or outpatient services; for example, by age or by sex. These are the kinds of data that are useful in bargaining with providers and in marketing.[12] Many health care insurers and providers now hire firms to analyze their paid claims to determine utilization of a particular benefit, help set prices, negotiate rates, and so forth.

Systems on the market today do not provide adequate data for setting sound premium rates or for determining utilization patterns. Managed care information systems should be able to accommodate multiple option plans and contract benefit variations, provide fast and accurate claims processing, and accommodate electronic claims transfer.[13]

In a recent survey by the Healthcare Financial Management Association, 65 percent of all respondents said today's information systems for managed care could not support management decision making. Over 50 percent cited these systems as the top challenge in setting up managed care operations.[14]

Potential Impact of New Technologies

New technologies such as image-based storage, image satellite transmission, and information integration (voice, data, image, text) are now being introduced into health care information systems; networks are being touted as "integrated" approaches by some vendors; medical expert systems are beginning to be used in ambulatory and hospital clinic settings to provide possible diagnoses and treatments for patients; and graphics, color, and windows are making automation more interesting and versatile even for the novice. The key question to be answered is whether or not vendors and providers will be able to effectively integrate these promising new technologies with their existing financial, administrative, and clinical systems while achieving tangible benefits and improving the quality of patient care.

Image-Based Storage and Information Integration

Breakthroughs in image-based storage (compact and Write-Once-Read-Many [WORM] optical disks) and in information integration (voice, data, text, and image) have the potential to revolutionize health care automation over the next five to ten years. This technology, properly used, could provide more timely, selective, or comprehensive information for the treatment of patients, at a relatively low cost.[15]

One example might be the (future) electronic ambulatory medical record integrated with radiology picture archiving and communications data, as well as with patient financial and administrative data, which could be instantaneously transmitted via satellite to a hospital 25 miles away for examination by a specialist.

Users would have to be able to index images in a variety of ways. Hardware and software architectures would have to treat images as data elements. Today, mismatched technologies, unmanageable volumes of data, and wasteful duplication reduce the ability of institutions to manage their strategic information. In the future, however, information and image management effectively integrated with other health care systems could give an institution a decided competitive edge.[16]

Tools for Information Resource Management

Decision support systems, artificial intelligence, expert systems, and knowledge-based systems have begun to play an important role in health care information systems. An on-line diagnostic expert system, DXplain, is now commercially available through the AMA/Net on-line service. This is a sophisticated decision support system that links observations and symptoms with associated diseases. Drawbacks include its inability to create causal relationships between symptoms and diseases, its lack of specialty information, and its limited vocabulary.

Eleven other medical expert systems were in use, in prototype, or in clinical testing in January 1988. All are standalone systems; none is integrated/interfaced with other systems.[17] Several health care vendors, including 3M, Cerner, Knowledge Data Systems, McDonnell Douglas, and Unisys, have announced experiments with expert systems.[18]

Expert and knowledge-based systems in health care are coming under increasing scrutiny as the Food and Drug Administration considers whether or not they are "medical devices" and therefore subject to extensive clinical testing prior to approval for general use.[19]

Open Architecture and Network Systems Integration

Many hardware and telecommunications vendors today are focusing on the development of shared communications protocols. The supporters of the Open Systems Interconnection (OSI) model of the International Standards Organization (ISO) have made significant progress over the last five years. Their aim is to have an environment in which products of multiple vendors with multiple architectures can more readily communicate. This is not going to happen overnight and will continue to require extensive investment in research and development by the major players. D.E.C. and IBM are reluctant and late participants in this process.[20-22]

Led by Donald Simborg, developer of STATLAN, and by Enterprise Systems, Inc., a group of software vendors and health care users (MEDIX) has been working to develop shared applications protocols for Health Level 7 (HL7) of the OSI model. Their approach is to define all of the standard protocols for admission/discharge/transfer (ADT), orders, results, and other discrete interfaces. It will be difficult for this group to reach consensus on a minimum data set, let alone the whole health care community. Major HIS vendors would also need to lend their support and invest heavily in research and development to accomplish this, an unlikely event.[23]

The Simborg system is a network systems integrator. Implementation is under way in several sites to provide synchronized transmissions of ADT, orders, and other key data to a host of disparate vendors' systems in minicomputer networks. This is an interesting approach, but it involves considerable redundancy and does not yet work completely anywhere, despite years of development.[24,25]

New Technologies: Promising but Unproven

Although these new technologies are exciting and offer promise, the probability of having proven, workable solutions available in the foreseeable future is extremely low. Experience in the health care computing industry over the past 20 years has shown this. A typical example is one in which a user of patient accounting and patient care or laboratory systems (from one or multiple vendors) has to install expensive network matrix switches with specialized software and protocol converters in order to avoid having two sets of incompatible terminals and printers (ASCII and IBM 3270-type devices) at each nursing station or in an admissions office. Another example is the bedside terminal, which has been talked about for at least ten years. A small number of vendors are now developing HIS systems that incorporate this technology, but today none are fully operational.

Progress, especially in health care, is slow. Since the inception of automated hospital information systems in the early 1960s, the health care industry has been plagued by a lack of objective information on the actual capabilities of vendor products. Some organizations, unable to assess their own needs realistically , have bought products based on exaggerated vendor claims of capabilities, and consequently have been unable to realize appropriate benefits from these systems.

Prospective buyers must be able to distinguish working systems and technologies from "vaporware." For information on specific vendors, see chapter 9 and also appendixes A and B.

Today No Products Fit Long-Term Needs

As alarming as it may sound, no products today fit the long-term needs of the ambulatory care information systems market or the health care market in general. Many lack key features and functions necessary for comprehensive automation of the work environment. The large number of vendors and products on the market makes it difficult for buyers to make informed decisions. In addition, vendors often lack a complete understanding of their clients' needs, the markets served, and the products available. Given this predicament, health care organizations need to recognize that their next set of computer replacement decisions will only meet some of their automation needs and therefore serve as an interim solution. Nonetheless, with realistic expectations health care organizations should continue to take advantage of automation by replacing systems when appropriate.

In an environment with multiple vendors and many products there are frequent incompatibilities, and information exchanges are costly, inefficient, error-prone, and sometimes ineffective. Integration is a concept, not a reality. So-called integrated products have little functionality and face future technical difficulties.

Networking is not the perfect short-term solution. It sounds promising and is being promoted by some vendors and do-it-yourself users, but there are many challenges, such as complex user interfaces, and costs are high.

Making Successful Purchases

Despite the problems inherent in many of the products available today, health care providers will continue to acquire new or replacement systems. Unfortunately, they are often disappointed with the computer systems they have purchased because they have unrealistic expectations about what computers can do for them, and because they do not fully understand what they need and what they have bought.

To be successful, plans and purchases must be based on accurate assessments of available software solutions, and on a thorough understanding of the marketplace. Buyers must adjust their expectations to more realistic levels. Chapters 4 and 5 cover assessing expectations and determining needs for computer systems in more detail.

The Health Care System of the Future

Vendors in the marketplace today are turning increasingly toward network-based solutions to the hospital corporations' desires for integration. The problem with this is that they are really addressing connectivity and interfacing issues, not true integration, where duplicate functions and redundant data entry and storage are eliminated and where information transfer/access takes place instantaneously. No one is doing this today because the technology is not there. It might not be possible to do this functionally within the software of multiple vendors' systems at any price because the commitment, the shared vision of the outcome, and the creativity to achieve this are currently missing.

When users talk about their desires for future systems, they talk about eliminating redundant data entry. They talk about having common registration so that patients are not registered at 10 locations during an ambulatory care visit group/encounter and so that the registration does not take place in six different systems with different aims and methods. Users also want an electronic medical record that captures information from all of the relevant episodes of care that make up the often-fragmented ambulatory care case. Furthermore, users talk about having a single source or approach for updating the patient's demographic and insurance data. They want consistency and accuracy. They also want all of the data elements they can possibly think of at any point in time available to them immediately, whether those data are billing and medical records data or nursing orders or mental health test results. They also do not want unauthorized persons to see or modify those data. Beyond this, a primary objective is to be able to buy any software package they need to extend their automated functions, and to integrate it effortlessly and inexpensively.

Response time on this future system should never concern the users. Above all, this system should be relatively inexpensive to operate, should eliminate the tons of paper that currently bury them, and should give them many analytic functions with which to manage their information resource. How this is done is of no concern to the users as long as it works.

Of course, no such system exists today, and probably will not exist for many years. When it does, the moral, ethical, and legal questions surrounding that ubiquitous data haven will be enormous.

Conclusion

What is the ultimate answer to users' dreams for better health care systems? It remains to be fully articulated and developed. Vendors and prospective users will need to collaborate and to invest heavily in this process in order to bring better, more comprehensive products to this market. In the meantime, users should continue to move forward, evaluating their needs realistically and understanding what they are buying. Multientity health care organizations will continue to set directions and priorities for new products as they continue to be the dominant investors in the ambulatory care and hospital information systems markets.

References

1. Steinwachs, D. M. Ambulatory care management information systems: future directions. *Journal of Ambulatory Care Management* May 1985, p. 91.

2. Cohen, M. R., and Hill, H. L. Key to successful hospital automation: realistic appraisal of needs and products. *HFMA First Illinois Speaks* Aug.–Sept. 1988, pp. 20, 29.

3. Dorenfest, S. I. Viewpoint: health care managers should capitalize on potential cost savings of automation. *Modern Healthcare* 18(28):49, July 8, 1988.

4. Dorenfest, S. I. *Business Opportunities in the Hospital Computer Market*. Northbrook, IL: Sheldon I. Dorenfest & Associates, June 1989, pp. 11–20.

5. Dorenfest, S. I. *Hospital Information Systems: State of the Art, 1988 ed*. Northbrook, IL: Sheldon I. Dorenfest & Associates, 1988.

6. Dorenfest, S. I. *Business Opportunities in the Hospital Computer Market*. Northbrook, IL: Sheldon I. Dorenfest & Associates, June 1989.

7. MacKay, J. M., and Lamb, C. W. Research in brief: tailoring hospital marketing efforts to physicians' needs. *Journal of Healthcare Marketing* 8(40):59, Dec. 1988.

8. MacKay and Lamb, p. 59.

9. Super, K. E. Hospitals ponder direct sales, physician marketing strategies. *Modern Healthcare* 17(1):68, Jan. 2, 1987.

10. MacKay and Lamb, p. 59.

11. Computer courses more common in medical schools. *National Report on Computers & Health* 9(15):6, July 25, 1988.

12. Survey reveals woeful data collection at HMOs. *National Report on Computers & Health* 9(16):5, Aug. 8, 1988.

13. Bona, G. M. HMO information system needs. *HealthWeek HCIS Outlook* Nov. 28, 1988, p. 21.

14. Survey finds information systems inadequate. *Healthcare Financial Management* 43(1):64, Jan. 1989.

15. Want, F. A. The promise and perils of information integration. *Computers in Healthcare* 8(14):30–31, Dec. 1987.

16. Want, pp. 30–31.

17. Batcha, B. Diagnosis with the touch of a finger. *Computerworld* Jan. 18, 1988, p. 64.

18. Childs, B. W. Artificial intelligence and expert systems. *U.S. Healthcare* 5(10):8–9, Oct. 1988.

19. Samuel, F. E., Jr. HIMA and the FDA. *HealthWeek HCIS Outlook* Nov. 28, 1988, p. 19.

20. Lockwood, R. Global networking unity. *Personal Computing* 12:34, Aug. 1988.

21. Sullivan, K. B. Demand for OSI is strong, yet hurdles remain. *PC Week* 5:8, Nov. 7, 1988.

22. Holmes, B. L. What's in store for networking standards? *Computers in Healthcare* 9(10):36–37, Oct. 1988.

23. Simborg, D. W. The case for the HL7 standard. *Computers in Healthcare* 9(1):39–42, Jan. 1988.

24. Children's goes beyond LAN to "virtual database." *National Report on Computers & Health* 9(24):1, 4, 5, Nov. 28, 1988.

25. Donald Simborg on LANs and Distributed Hospital Computing, pp. 5–6.

Chapter 4

Improved Management through Automation

Walter C. Zerrenner

Information Systems Management: The Needs Gap

As health care business needs have increased, the gap between those needs and information systems performance has gotten even wider. The focus of information systems has changed from improving internal operating efficiency to directly delivering products or services to the health care system.

Targeting information systems to business needs means emphasizing effectiveness over efficiency wherever possible. It means raising technology sufficient for the need. It means providing delivery systems for sustainable competitive advantage. Today's information systems must meet the needs of all types of health care managers, particularly for the emerging ambulatory care professional. The key is the interpretation of data as *information* that can be used to make sound decisions.

This chapter, written from a broad management perspective, first reviews the traditional systems approach to meeting management information needs and explains why it is no longer appropriate. Specific information needs of ambulatory care systems and critical success factors are then discussed. The last part of the chapter describes technological advances that are becoming important tools in the management of ambulatory care patients.

Traditional Systems Approach—It Does Not Work Any More

The traditional approach to meeting "management information needs" is to produce tons of reports that contain all the information anyone could possibly want. A review of how information systems have evolved provides a good perspective for examining the challenges faced by today's information systems.

The term *management information systems (MIS)* has over the years come to mean the accounting and transaction processing systems that are the backbone of most health care financial systems. Out of these systems come reports that summarize transactions and financial conditions for management review. Management information systems now symbolize corporate computing, and in most managers' eyes they are simply data processing. They are characterized by large centralized data bases and are justified on the basis of cost savings resulting from the automation of clerical and accounting functions. These systems tend to be large in scope, highly specialized, and batch-oriented. Interactive functions in the MIS environment have been primarily the keying in of transaction data, as opposed to on-line information retrieved by managers.

The era of corporate computing was characterized by a focus on tactical instead of strategic systems. The traditional technology involved high-performance systems with long development cycles. In an attempt to address strategic information needs, the industry moved to the era of individual computing.

With the advent of the personal computer, individual computing proliferated rapidly. Personal computers (PCs) were favored over time-sharing bureaus because the low computing functions were powerful, easy to learn, and inexpensive. Additionally, microcomputers that were able to run similar applications with even greater number-crunching horsepower began to appear.

Individual computing fell short in the effort to address strategic systems and senior management needs. The characteristic of these systems was that they were analytical in nature. Individual computing functions made their biggest impact not as information systems but as analytical, decision-simulation tools for solving a range of ad hoc problems.

As the earlier generations of corporate computing and individual computing were commercialized, managers tended to adopt the technology first and then tried to figure out what to do with it. In today's business world that approach is grossly inadequate. Today's technology is more powerful, more diverse, and more entwined with health care's critical success factors. Management cannot merely react to new technology but must be responsive to it in correlation with the changing business environment.

Management Expectations

At a major health care company in Chicago, the chief financial officer vents a frustration with computers. "I don't want any computer terminals in my office. I already get more reports than I need. Most of my managers have PCs in their offices, but they aren't used much because staff analysts work the numbers and the secretaries do all the typing. The information systems people seem bright enough, but they have a hard time understanding what I need. I want reports that save time. I am not impressed by massive amounts of data."

Sound familiar? The words may vary but in health care businesses everywhere, there are managers who are information users, not analysts. These managers set policy and make decisions—they are not the staff who execute those decisions. The notion that every manager's and executive's desk needs to be equipped with an intelligent workstation ignores the very essence of their jobs. Managers want to review relevant information so that they can formulate decisions and action plans. They need improved access to information that lets them carry out their decision-making responsibilities. This requirement is not filled by word processing, spreadsheets, or integrated software packages.

Examples of information needed to make sound decisions might include the following:

- Clear presentation of clinical findings to prevent oversight
- Possible diagnosis and appropriate procedures
- Options for lower-cost drugs and other supplies
- Existing practice patterns within the ambulatory care setting
- Cost-per-visit comparisons with competitive care centers
- Research/use of tests/experiments

Management must identify information needs and critical success factors; they must eliminate the information systems constraints in the organization that make it difficult to achieve their objectives.

Management must come to grips with the fact that the traditional approach cannot turn out effective systems in short time frames. Strategic systems are critical to the success of even the most promising health care business. Responsibility for this issue can no longer be delegated to the lower levels of management. Senior management must become directly involved in planning, implementing, and managing those applications that address the organization's goals. Managers must select strategic applications that are accurately focused on the true critical success factors that contribute to organizational goals.

The Value of Strategic Information Systems

Strategic information systems are those that could conceivably determine an organization's survival by enhancing services while continuing to reduce costs. Managers must control unreimbursable products and services and provide the necessary documentation to ensure adequate payment. The business needs cannot be supplied on the basis of information from a single isolated source.

Strategic systems are those that will provide an organization with the ability to add value to its products and services. This added value could be transformed into higher profit margins and potentially greater market share. Sometimes just having the right information on hand can be strategic.

Management needs to take a hard look at the organization's current information systems projects and ask appropriate questions of them:

- Are they mission-critical?
- Will they make a difference in the success of the business?
- Will they affect the way the organization does business?

Today's senior managers should be concerned with two issues: (1) identifying strategic opportunities for the organization and (2) getting information systems implemented fast.

Data Rich, Information Poor

In order to identify strategic opportunities and implement methods of attaining them, managers need to look at the way information is gathered. The aforementioned proliferation of comprehensive reports for management has resulted in an unprecedented explosion of printout. These reports fail, however, because by attempting to do all things for all people, they are virtually of no use to anyone. Many of these reports move directly from the computer room to the trash can. In addition to wasting computer resources and supplies, searching through all these data for that precious information is a costly process. Try building a three-year patient mix trend from 36 months of ADT reports!

What most information systems do not do is search for the relevant data and then turn them into meaningful information. Presentation of the data is equally important. It can include ratios, historical perspectives, comparisons, and other internal or external data and can be presented in meaningful form; for example, in tables, bar graphs, or scatter graphs.

To avoid being data rich and information poor, put information compression to work for you. Follow the 80/20 principle; that is, you can meet 80 percent of the business needs with 20 percent of the information. Identify which 20 percent of the information is the most important, and then make it easy for management to access the information. Management should have the easiest access to the most needed information. If access is provided to everything, the system will become too complicated and a fundamental objective of simplification will be overlooked.

Case Mix System Needs

Case mix refers to categories of patients in an institution at a given time who are classified by disease, procedure, method of payment, or other characteristics. Case mix systems will need to provide product-based financial and quality assurance information required by the ambulatory care decision makers. In order to control costs in this dynamic environment, providers must be able to predict and measure patterns of resource utilization by patient and must accurately identify and isolate costs with specific services. Although much of this valuable information can come from comparisons and reviews, it is always after the fact: the health care has been delivered, the costs have been incurred, and the patient has been discharged.

A critical capability of any case mix system is the ability to identify, segregate, and describe product and patient characteristics. The ideal system will need to provide real-time interaction with all types of health care professionals and management, drawing on their collective expertise for clinical and financial decisions. By combining detailed patient information with clinical protocols, health care delivery can be influenced at the time of prescription. This is accomplished through the use of information management tools such as decision support systems and expert systems technology, which are discussed later in this chapter.

Consequently, the effective use of decision support systems or expert systems technology can give providers a means to measure productivity and ensure efficiency in managing patient care. Regardless of what case mix classification is adopted, providers will be able to work effectively within their clinical, financial, and operational boundaries.

Information Systems in the 1990s

Much of the technology that will give managers the freedom to shape their organization is already commercialized, that is, expert systems and executive information systems. Expert and knowledge-based systems are rapidly appearing in business settings. Many of the major Fortune 500 companies have at least one production system using this technology. Executive information systems, which track both internal and external information, enable management to control and monitor large, complex organizations.

In the early 1990s, these technologies will be widely used by most major corporations and by sophisticated health care organizations. Management will be able to pick and choose applications that fit their requirements. Computers will be faster, smaller, more reliable, and easier to use. Computers will store vast amounts of information, and they will be flexible enough to allow organizations to change their information and communication systems as the environment changes. Management will not only react to technology but will use it to shape the organization.

Decision Support Systems/Expert Technology

Decision support systems are designed to enhance the decision-making process. Every decision has two major factors that determine its effectiveness: (1) how much do you know about the situation when you make the decision? and (2) how long does it take to make the decision and take action? Making decisions in the absence of information, "winging it," is usually the result of having too little time to gather useful supporting data. Winging it is risky, so managers tend to learn as much as possible before making a decision and quickly reach a point of diminishing returns.

Decisions must be timely. Many managers are guilty of studying problems to death. They theorize that if delayed long enough, the decision becomes meaningless, and management is thereby protected against the embarrassment of a bad decision. Thus, the time value of decision making is lost.

Considering that decisions lose their effectiveness with time and that too much study yields diminishing returns, there must be an optimum time to make a decision. Effective managers recognize this and maintain a balance between insight and timeliness. The overall effectiveness of the decision-making process is improved by speeding up the manager's learning process—precisely the function of expert technology.

Health care expert systems contain collections of known facts covering areas of medical knowledge, reimbursement criteria, and the cost of care. These facts reflect the thinking process of experts in the health care industry. In expert systems, the decision-making process is created and modified by management and qualified professionals, not by the system itself.

Expert systems contain a knowledge base that is a collection of clinical criteria, protocols, and rules defined by the health care organization. Expert systems support health care delivery at the point of care and offer management timely assistance for making informed decisions. Rather than just reporting data, they derive logical conclusions about the information.

Given the complex protocols and rules required in a health care setting and the enormous amount of data required, the health care industry is a natural environment for decision support systems and the usefulness of expert technology.

Executive Information Systems

Whereas typical information systems have served the clerical and accounting functions and decision support systems have provided analytical tools, executive information systems (EIS) solve a range of ad hoc problems. Executive information systems serve management whose job it is to review operating numbers, budgets, project progress reports, market survey data, and countless what-if scenarios.

The EIS user does not manipulate data; members of the staff perform that function. The EIS user is the policymaker rather than the executor of policy. He or she has responsibility to ensure that organizational objectives are achieved. This is the link between critical success factors (CSF) and EIS. The EIS data base contains the information necessary to support management's control of the CSF process.

Executive information systems have characteristics that distinguish them from other established software product areas for information systems and decision support systems. They are aimed at managers who currently have few if any computer-based systems to assist them with their day-to-day responsibilities. They bring together relevant data from a number of internal and external sources and deliver the information to the user quickly and in a meaningful way. Unlike traditional systems that focus on data storage, EIS focus on the retrieval of information. The emphasis is on reducing the number of logical decisions that the user must make in order to obtain useful information.

Executive information systems are just starting to emerge in health care organizations. There are two principal reasons why it has taken so long for EIS to be accepted. The first is cost. All health care organizations have established cost containment as a critical success factor. Therefore, any EIS must be economically viable, based on the value it provides to users relative to cost. The second reason is ease of use. If management is to accept the use of computers in their daily activities, these systems must be productive and easy to use.

The aspect of technology that has paved the way for EIS is the proliferation of interactive operating systems and the ability of personal computers to communicate with mainframe computers. Cost, ease of use, speed, and responsiveness are crucial in the success of an executive information system. As a result of the dramatic reduction in cost of EIS, the advancements in software, and the increasing awareness of the importance of high-quality, timely information to major clinical and financial issues, EIS will proliferate rapidly in the health care industry in the next several years.

SURROUND^{SM} Technology

The typical health care environment is a mainframe-based centralized information system that runs patient accounting and other financial applications. Clinical systems are normally supplied by niche vendors and run on departmental computers. These systems are installed in a stand-alone manner and serve specialized information needs. There is a lack of integration among these various health care applications, and yet an integrated clinical and financial data base is essential in order to manage health care costs and optimize medical resources. Until now, no vendor has developed applications serving every clinical and financial area, nor have vendors solved the problem of connecting computer systems within and between health care facilities.

One approach to connecting divergent computer applications involves surrounding the existing systems with a much more flexible and functional system. This approach is appropriately called the SURROUND[SM] architecture, developed by the Cambridge Technology Group, Inc.

Users of the SURROUND system interact only with SURROUND, which then interacts with the other systems to get the information needed. The user decides which of the existing systems will be surrounded and what information should be retrieved. This approach is reportedly implemented in a relatively short time frame because it does not require the rebuilding of the older applications. External systems can also be accessed by the SURROUND system, allowing users to integrate external with internal information for strategic purposes.

Distributed Processing/Networks

The personal computer has been well accepted by organizations, and health care is no exception. The most significant challenge facing organizations will be the networking of personal computers, minicomputers, and mainframes with each other and one another. There is a technology trend toward bedside terminals and intelligent workstations that have access to clinical data bases. Health care facilities are considering local network technology as the link for distributed processing.

Local area networks (LANs) are emerging as the preferred approach for the sharing of information among departmental systems.

Supporting a variety of computer applications running on divergent computers presents substantial compatibility problems. To deal with this obstacle, several communication standards for the health care industry have emerged. These standards are intended to simplify the task of networking computer systems within and between health care facilities. Two of these standards are Health Level 7 (HL7) and the IEEP157 Medical Data Exchange (MEDIX). Both of these rely on Open Systems Interconnection (OSI) protocols.

These efforts will allow the users to protect their investment in application architecture, hardware, and software. Many application software vendors have already committed to standard interfaces. Health care facilities may be geographically dispersed, but information and communication systems will enable users with complementary skills to work together.

Technology in the 21st Century

Although current computer technology lags behind the needs of most users, in the 21st century, personal computers will be as powerful as today's supercomputers. They will be able to store vast amounts of information, and they will be flexible enough to allow organizations to change their information and communication systems as the technological environment changes. The supercomputers will run at speeds a thousand times faster than today's. Computer chips will have more than one billion elements, compared with one million now.

Health care organizations will be able to communicate voluminous amounts of information in a variety of forms (data, text, image, voice, and video) over long distances within seconds. Improved reliability and security will support the faster network speeds and improved systems performance. Plugging computers into networks will be as easy as plugging in your telephone today. Telephones will be replaced by computer phones that will convert speech into text and transmit images, voices, and data simultaneously.

Organizations will no longer be restricted to keyboard entry. Voice recognition technology will allow users to dictate messages and create and revise text as easily as using a dictaphone. Physicians and nurses wearing lapel microphones will be updating patient charts and medical records as they talk.

As computers become faster at processing and communicating information, companies will need ways to control and manage the technology. Optical storage media will be used to store and retrieve more information networks, which will do away with the rigid static data bases in use today.

By the 21st century, health care companies will routinely use expert systems and knowledge-based applications. Knowledge bases, which contain both logic and data, will be commonplace. Technology will be used more than ever in tasks requiring judgment and expert knowledge. Technologies will be well developed to meet the needs of health care executives. Computers and software will support executive planning, decision making, communication, and control activities.

Management's Future Role

The next decade will see new technologies proliferate throughout thousands of organizations. The vast majority of managers will have PCs on their desks, which will provide them with most of their day-to-day information needs. Computers will be efficient and flexible enough to allow each manager to adjust an information system to his or her own management style. Technology will be applied on a broad scale dealing with issues directly relating to management.

The integration of mainframe and microcomputer technologies has opened the way to a new generation of information technology that managers can relate to. Information systems managers who learn and understand business concepts such as critical success factors and information compression will be able to spearhead the introduction of information technology into the executive suite. The evidence is growing that the strategic use of information by managers will be the most deciding competitive business factor in the decade ahead. The managers who make this happen and promote new technologies will realize a new status in their organization.

It is clearly time for managers to get off the technology sideline and get involved. Senior executives are increasingly feeling the need to become informed, energized, and engaged in information systems.

The Information Systems Executive

In order for the information systems executive to address future technologies, he or she must be repositioned in the organization. The organizational restructuring of the information systems function requires the integration of telecommunications and information processing. This is necessary to support the information gathering and dissemination for addressing the mainstream information needs of the organization. Successful information systems executives will have a well-defined perspective on information systems technology and a clear vision of where their health care organizations should be going with that technology.

The information systems executive will be an aggressive, proactive, communication-oriented executive who focuses heavily on helping the organization adapt to a changing technical environment. This executive will ensure that rapidly evolving technical opportunities are understood, planned for, and implemented in the organization. The top information systems executive will be a thinker, a planner, and a coordinator rather than the traditional implementer and doer.

Conclusion

Using exciting technological advancements alone will not guarantee success in meeting ambulatory care information needs. Other guidelines for success include the following:

- Use strategic information systems that will enhance your institution's competitive position.
- Get senior management involved in planning, implementing, and managing applications that meet the institution's goals.
- Target which information you need to meet most of your goals and make it easy to access; discard the rest.

Chapter 5

Assessing Needs and Examining Options

Erica L. Drazen

This chapter will demonstrate the process of determining information systems needs as a prelude to examining various ways to obtain computer systems. The advantages and drawbacks of each option, as well as a method for comparing the risks, will be described.

Asking the Right Question

The most important step in examining the options for information systems in ambulatory care is asking the correct question. The question is not "What computer system should I buy?" It is not even "Should I buy a computer system?" Instead, the correct question is "How can I manage information to meet my needs better?"

There are two important elements to this question. First, any decision about information systems must be driven by your needs—not by what your competitors are buying or what vendors say you must have. The second element is the objective of improved information management, not acquisition of computer systems. Once needs are identified, the best solution may include improvements in any of the following: manual systems, telecommunications systems, or computer systems. All three options must be considered when determining your best solution.

Assessing Needs

Needs assessment is key to improving management, and it could fill an entire chapter. This chapter touches on some of its elements.

Although it is true that efforts spent in assessing needs pay off in terms of better decisions, it is also possible to spend too much time and effort in this activity. As a rule, 10 percent of the amount of money you are willing to spend on improvements should be spent on assessing needs. If a needs assessment has not been done for a long time, the requirement may be slightly higher. At this level of finding, it is not possible to do a "bottom-up" assessment involving an examination of all your business and patient care processes; however, usually 80 percent of the needs (usually more than you have budget to address) can be identified using one of several "top-down" techniques. (A "bottom-up" approach means assessing all processes in detail; it is a micro-level approach that would be very time-consuming. A "top-down" approach means assessing your needs from a more global [macro] level and delving into detail only when necessary.)

Identifying Information Issues within Your Practice

Looking at trends and conducting staff interviews and surveys should result in a consensus of important issues that should be addressed by a new information system.

Trend Analyses

Trend analyses can be done simply by analyzing performance indicators and comparing current to past performance (for example, on a monthly or annual basis). Information gleaned from a trend analysis can be incorporated into the decision-making process so that more-informed decisions and assessments can be made.

Trend analyses of key indicators will show where performance has changed over time. Are payments becoming slower? Are bills getting out later? Are more patients not keeping appointments? Are patients switching to other physicians? Positive responses to these questions may indicate problems. If you cannot obtain information to evaluate any of these indicators, this in itself identifies a management need for information.

A trend analysis will indicate how well your organization is doing relative to the past, but you also want to know how it is performing in absolute terms. The best way to do this is by comparison with national norms. Where there are no national norms, you must obtain available information on the competition, perhaps by asking newer staff members how your organization's performance compares with their past settings.

Interviews

Staff interviews, if well managed, also can identify high-priority problems. Interviews are more useful when they are conducted by an outside, independent third party. (In internal interviews there is a great temptation to say what the interviewer wants to hear.) The focus of the interviews has to be on high-priority problems, or else you will create a long "wish list" and promote unrealistic expectations.

You can focus on high-priority needs by asking questions such as, "What are the two areas where you believe departmental operations (or your practice) need to improve?" or "What could be the most important future change to your department and what will you need to manage it successfully?"

Drawing conclusions from interview data depends on the interview. Sometimes the interview is worthless; that's why you often interview several people. Other times the interview provides tremendous insight into problem areas and potential solutions.

Surveys

Staff surveys can serve two purposes. They can confirm or prioritize information on problem areas identified on performance reviews or interviews, or they can elicit new issues. Satisfaction surveys can be conducted with all "customers": physician staff, patients, and insurers (or other payers). Areas of dissatisfaction among these customers indicate issues for further investigation. A sample survey questionnaire is shown in figure 5-1.

Analyzing the Root Cause

Once issues have been identified, they need to be translated into solutions. To do this, one must identify the root cause of each problem— otherwise you will treat symptoms rather than core problems. For example, if you have discovered that patients are very dissatisfied with their access to appointments and are seeking care elsewhere, this does not necessarily mean that a computerized patient appointment system would solve the problem. To find the root cause and come up with effective solutions, you need to ask a series of questions. In this case, here are some questions you would ask:

- Why are patients dissatisfied with access to appointments? (Possible answer: because they often reach a busy signal when calling.)
- Why do they reach a busy signal? (Possible answer: because there are only two lines coming into the appointment area or because everyone calls between 9 and 10 a.m.)

The answers to these questions should yield some needs that can be addressed. For example, a telephone upgrade could provide more incoming capacity (assuming that staff members are available to answer additional calls); appointment hours could be extended to avoid peaks; or patients could be encouraged during a visit to book return appointments.

Figure 5-1. Sample Survey Questionnaire

Your answers to the following questions will provide insight into the performance of your
organization's current information systems. Please indicate your satisfaction with each item as it
relates to your outpatient practice by marking an X in the column that best describes your opinion.

Please rate your satisfaction:	Very Satisfied	Somewhat Satisfied	Neutral	Somewhat Dissatisfied	Very Dissatisfied
a. Availability of outpatient records at time of patient visit	1. _____	2. _____	3. _____	4. _____	5. _____
b. Availability of outpatient records for telephone consults	1. _____	2. _____	3. _____	4. _____	5. _____
c. Completeness of clinical information in outpatient records	1. _____	2. _____	3. _____	4. _____	5. _____
d. Accuracy of test results	1. _____	2. _____	3. _____	4. _____	5. _____
e. Legibility of elements in outpatient records	1. _____	2. _____	3. _____	4. _____	5. _____
f. Time it takes to locate information in outpatient records	1. _____	2. _____	3. _____	4. _____	5. _____
g. Ease of ordering laboratory tests	1. _____	2. _____	3. _____	4. _____	5. _____
h. Turnaround time for STAT laboratory test results	1. _____	2. _____	3. _____	4. _____	5. _____
i. Turnaround time for routine laboratory test results	1. _____	2. _____	3. _____	4. _____	5. _____
j. Ease of ordering radiology procedures	1. _____	2. _____	3. _____	4. _____	5. _____
k. Turnaround time for STAT radiology reports	1. _____	2. _____	3. _____	4. _____	5. _____
l. The process for notifying you about abnormal laboratory test results	1. _____	2. _____	3. _____	4. _____	5. _____
m. The process for notifying you about abnormal radiology reports	1. _____	2. _____	3. _____	4. _____	5. _____
n. Time you spend locating test results	1. _____	2. _____	3. _____	4. _____	5. _____
o. Availability of outpatient medication profiles	1. _____	2. _____	3. _____	4. _____	5. _____
p. Completeness of outpatient medication profiles	1. _____	2. _____	3. _____	4. _____	5. _____
q. Availability of information on medication allergies	1. _____	2. _____	3. _____	4. _____	5. _____
r. Availability of information about inpatient care at the time of the outpatient visit	1. _____	2. _____	3. _____	4. _____	5. _____

Root cause analysis will lead to a list of needs that then can be translated into effective solutions.

Setting Priorities

Addressing all the root causes of the high-priority issues still may exceed the budget; it usually also exceeds the practice's ability to accept change. Therefore, priorities must be set. Setting priorities involves the following:

- *Analyzing the importance of the underlying issue to the practice.* Is it necessary for survival? Will it contribute to short- and long-term revenues? Will it address a critical patient care issue?
- *Studying cost and feasibility.* Some solutions may be inexpensive (for example, using an existing computer capability no one knew existed). Others may be quite expensive. The level of risk involved in each project also will differ.
- *Examining leverage.* Fixing some root causes may address several issues and, therefore, those should receive higher priority over root causes that affect only one issue.

After projects that receive good ratings on all criteria are selected, the next step is to assign a weight to each factor. The weight given to each factor is a practice decision that will affect the priorities.

Examining System Options

If the needs analysis leads to a conclusion that a computer system is the most effective way to solve a high-priority problem, the next step involves choosing among computer system options. The traditional options considered when buying a computer system were "build" or "buy." An implicit choice always has been "wait and see." In today's cost-control environment, "make do" should be on everyone's list. For ambulatory care, another option may be to "borrow" from a local hospital or HMO. Most of these options can be pursued singly or in combination. They vary in terms of cost, fit with your needs, and probability of success.

Build

A few hospitals chose to build computer software during the past decade. This also was the dominant solution in the early days of HMOs. Building results in higher costs and higher risks to achieving success within planned costs and schedules. In theory, building leads to greater satisfaction of your needs. You can specify how each function will work and customize the system to fit your practice. There are now only two situations where the benefits outweigh the risks and would lead to a build strategy:

- *When your needs are unique and not addressed by any existing products.* HMOs developed their own systems because hospital and physician office systems did not meet their needs.
- *When you are committed to a research program to advance the state of the art.* Several teaching hospitals have developed their own computer systems, which have advanced the state of art both in financial and patient care applications. This has been less common among ambulatory practices because they rarely have the staff to develop systems.

Most ambulatory care practices will find that their needs are met by existing systems, and few will have the clinical and information systems staff to devote to developing new applications. Therefore, it would be rare to find an ambulatory care practice that could support a build strategy or a practice where the promise of better functions would outweigh the risks.

A compromise to building is a "buy–build" strategy conducted in collaboration with a vendor. In this strategy, you would buy a set of applications from one vendor and agree to collaborate on enhancing them or on building new ones. Because there are more customers than vendors, this option is not always open, but it certainly is worth pursuing over a straight-build strategy. A collaboration takes advantage of the functional expertise and operating environment of the user and the technical and development skills of the vendor.

One major risk in a buy–build strategy is that the vendor will withdraw support. The risk is less likely if the application has wide market potential, if the vendor is committed to ambulatory care systems, if the vendor is financially stable, and if an explicit contract has been written between you and the vendor.

Another risk is that once software is developed, your organization will become a demonstration site for potential customers. Although you may not mind at first, a steady stream of visitors can be disruptive. Limits must be negotiated when a contract is signed for development.

Buy

A buy strategy has been the one most frequently pursued in ambulatory care (and hospital) settings. Many vendors have developed systems of varying sophistication and costs. Most needs will be well served by these systems. A buy strategy will involve lower risk to costs, schedules, and functions than a build strategy—although some compromises will be made between the ideal and the available functions.

Within a buy system, there are two choices—a single-vendor solution or a multiple-vendor solution. Buying from a single vendor increases the likelihood that the applications will be integrated and requires less management time than a multiple-vendor plan, which requires time to resolve issues among vendors on roles and responsibilities.

However, because there are numerous niche vendors with highly specialized products (cost accounting, oncology practice management, and so forth), buying from several vendors will increase the number of specific needs you will be able to address. A multiple-vendor strategy will be successful if it is implemented within an overall technical computer strategy to ensure that the systems will work together. It also requires strong project management.

It usually is preferable to choose one prime vendor who can meet most of your needs and then to pursue options where that prime vendor will interface with other specialty systems you want to add.

Wait and See

A wait and see strategy always has been one implicit strategy, and it is frequently an excuse for not automating. Usually it is evolving technology that is used to justify waiting and seeing. The rationale may be that "costs will come down with the next generation," "vendor X is about to introduce the perfect system," "we are awaiting a truly fault-tolerant system," or "we want a real fourth-generation language."

It is difficult to think of a situation where waiting would be preferable to solving the problems identified in a focused needs analysis. If you can wait, the application probably does not belong on your priority list. If it is on your priority list, you cannot afford to wait.

It always will be true that the next-generation system will have a better price/performance ratio, will be faster, will store more, and will have other desirable characteristics. However, today's systems are adequate, and waiting is rarely necessary. It is important to avoid buying an obsolete product; you must review both the technology and company as thoroughly as you would evaluate the functions provided by any system. For example, a vendor may announce a "new and improved" product, although it still sells an "older" product. If you are thinking about purchasing the older product, it is helpful to know how much the vendor still supports the older product. Vendors may not allocate much research and development investment for enhancements for older product lines.

Planning for the future (that is, the "see" part of wait and see) should be part of the examination of options. All products will need to be replaced, and planning for replacement should be part of the decision-making process.

Make Do

To get the most out of dollars spent on automation, you should maximize the use of your installed base of systems before considering other options. There are several reasons why this strategy is not often examined:

- *Looking to existing systems to do more may imply that they are currently poorly managed.* Because the current information manager is often a key player in examining options, it is natural that the issue of possible mismanagement is not raised. An objective outside party will probably be needed to look at the option of getting more out of existing systems.
- *Getting more out of existing systems requires technical expertise.* It is much more likely that technical limitations (rather than totally unused capabilities) are inhibiting a system's effectiveness. The system may need to be "tuned" to increase capacity, or perhaps a network is needed to enable disparate systems to provide integrated access to end users. Maybe PCs could be added to overcome limitations in ad hoc reporting capabilities of existing systems. Having the technical expertise to examine these types of options is a rarity in an ambulatory care setting.
- *Examining options often is supported by system vendors or consultants who may sell either systems or installation support services.* Both groups have a natural bias toward options that involve new systems. Both may offer excellent (and inexpensive) advice regarding the options, but those benefits must be weighed against possible prejudices against make-do options that may be in your best interests.
- *Supporting a "make-do" position is not very glamorous.* On an excitement scale, build comes first, then buy, then make do. Combined with the need to question management and confront technical issues, the make-do option becomes fairly low on a scale of fun things to do.

Still, the make-do option is realistic because of its low cost. Not only should it be the lowest in capital cost (because you salvage as much of your installed base as possible), but more important, it will involve the least commitment of staff time in conversion of data, in learning new systems, and in maintaining parallel operations.

When examining the ability of an existing system to meet needs, one rarely finds that all needs can be met via system enhancements or better use of the system capabilities. In most cases, a combined make-do and buy option will be selected. System upgrades or new applications may be purchased; or specialized systems may be purchased to run parallel to, or be interfaced with, existing systems.

When examining this option, make sure that the life-cycle costs of upgrading do not exceed the savings in purchase price and conversion. This risk is particularly high if you are working with old technology or with a system that has been abandoned by its vendor. Making do will not be an option if your technology is truly obsolete or if it is no longer supported by the system's vendor.

Borrow

Ambulatory care practices sometimes can borrow information systems from hospitals and possibly from HMOs. This has been an option for ambulatory care practices affiliated with hospitals, and it is now an option for most ambulatory practices. Hospitals are seeking to tie-in physicians and view information systems as a way to make that tie. Many of the clinical functions are the same within the two settings, and many hospitals have the capabilities to support their ambulatory care practices. Because the peak work load in inpatient and outpatient care tends to occur at different times, the hospital may have the capacity to support an ambulatory care setting.

One benefit of borrowing is that you will be acquiring a system that has been tested in your environment, with local expertise to call on if there are problems. The hospital, seeing other payoffs, may be willing to give you a good price for services. Another benefit is that by using the hospital's computer system, you could gain access to information about your hospitalized patients.

The biggest risk associated with borrowing a computer is that the lender is not necessarily business-oriented and may not have evaluated accurately the ability to provide services. You also need to be assured that the hospital will not have unauthorized access to data from your practice.

Summary of the Risks of Various Strategies

Table 5-1 presents a summary of the risks inherent in various strategies. To permit comparison, all issues have been stated negatively so that a high score indicates a risky decision. Ratings were based on a scale of 1 (no cost/risk) to 7 (very high cost/risk). The categories that were rated included:

Table 5-1. Example of Risks of Various Strategies

Type of Risk	Build	Buy—One Vendor	Buy—Multiple Vendor	Wait and See	Make-Do	Borrow
Unsatisfied needs	NA	4	2	6	3	4
Functional risk	6	2	2	NA	2	2
Technical risk	4	2	4	NA	4	3
Schedule risk	6	1	2	NA	2	4
Price	6	4	4	NA	1	2
Risk of costs exceeding plan	6	1	2	NA	2	2
Financial resources for implementation	3	4	3	NA	1	4
Level of project management	7	2	6	NA	2	4
Information systems expertise	7	2	4	NA	3	4

Note: The hypothetical results are based on a scale from 1 (no cost/risk) to 7 (very high cost/risk).

- *Unsatisfied needs:* The probability that the option you decide on will not meet all of your stated needs.
- *Functional risk:* The risk that the functions you expect from the system will not be delivered or will not work when they arrive.
- *Technical risk:* The risk that technically poor performance (lack of integration, poor response time, excessive downtime) will interfere with the system benefits.
- *Schedule risk:* The risk that the schedule for implementing systems will slip. The consequences are a longer time frame to achieve benefits.
- *Price risk:* The cost risk of acquiring the capabilities, either through development or outright purchase.
- *Excessive costs risk:* The probability that project costs will exceed plan.
- *Financial resources for implementation:* The risk that resources for training, duplicate work effort, conversion, and actual implementation of the system will not be available.
- *Level of project management:* The probability that the required level of project management expertise (in-house or acquired) will not be available.
- *Information systems expertise:* The level of information systems expertise (in-house or acquired) required for success.

The actual "score" any strategy will receive will depend on the specific option being considered. For example, all categories of risk would be high for a vendor just entering the market. It is also likely that the weights assigned to some categories will vary according to the practices' individual situation. For example, most practices will weigh "percentage of needs unsatisfied" higher than other categories because all needs being considered are high priority. Depending on the amount of money available, purchase price might be weighed higher or lower than other considerations. In the unusual case where all categories are weighed equally, the best scores would be achieved by the make-do and buy-from-one-vendor options. Major trade-offs among these alternatives are the high cost of the buy-from-vendor option versus the technical expertise required to achieve success with a make-do strategy.

Buying from multiple vendors and borrowing would be the next-best options. The multiple-vendor option would be more costly and more difficult to manage, but it would result in greater satisfaction of needs and less risk in adhering to a schedule.

As discussed previously, wait and see is not an applicable strategy for meeting urgent information management needs. The build option has the highest negative score mainly because of schedule, functional, and cost risk.

Looking toward Implementation

The experience gained in examining options will be helpful in the implementation process. You will learn whether or not you have an effective information management function within your institution. Some tests of the strength of the information management function are the following:

- Was there a logical candidate to head up the process of assessing needs and examining options?
- Was the logical candidate considered too valuable in his or her role as an information manager to devote to the project?
- Could someone answer questions such as:
  - How long does it take a request for a system change to be implemented?
  - What reports are used to manage day-to-day operations; what data are used in planning?
  - What was the last request for information that could not be satisfied?
  - How do our maintenance costs compare with industry averages?
  - Did managers, clinical and technical, cooperate with and respect the person designated as manager of the planning processes?

If the answer to all these questions is yes, then you probably have an effective information function within your organization. Any negative answers indicate that information management needs to be strengthened before implementing any changes. Selection and implementation will require more management than the needs assessment steps. Formalizing responsibility for information management will be critical to your future success.

Conclusion

To achieve the goal of better information management, managers must assess information gathered through trend analyses, interviews, and surveys in a way that addresses the root cause of problems. A careful examination of priorities will help ambulatory care managers decide whether build, buy, wait and see, make do, or borrow is the best strategy to meet their particular needs.

Chapter 6

System Evaluation and Implementation Strategies

Robert J. Feldman

This chapter presents strategies for evaluating the various vendor systems, selecting a system that best meets the institution's needs within identified constraints, and then implementing the selected system. The process of selecting and implementing an information system is greatly affected by the organization's operational, financial, and political environment. Each factor must be fully evaluated before a specific approach is chosen. This approach is applicable for all segments of the health care industry, including ambulatory care.

Developing a Plan

Before starting the process of selecting an information system, the institution must first review the specific goals for automation that were set as part of the needs assessment. Senior management should carefully examine their reasons for automation to help determine the appropriate group of vendors to evaluate. For example, is the system being installed to improve operational efficiency and productivity? Is the system being installed to improve patient care and the public image of the institution? Alternatively, is the system being installed to improve management reporting?

The second step is to determine which applications will be needed and what integration among applications is required. Appropriate constraints should also be considered at this time. Such constraints might include types of hardware the system would require or cost limitations. The institution should determine its ultimate goal in computerization so that the approach selected does not limit future options or restrict future systems growth.

The next step is to evaluate the current software and hardware environment. Most health care institutions have already computerized many applications. Unless the foundation is very weak, first consideration should be given to building upon the present approach to accomplish the institution's longer-term objectives. A complete inventory of software applications and computer equipment should be documented. With this information, information systems management will be able to determine which hardware will be usable in the new configuration and which applications not being replaced will need to be converted.

Organizing Internal Resources

An effective organization that seeks the support of potential users and management is critical to the future success of the automation effort. Committees provide a convenient mechanism to bring involved parties together during both the selection and the implementation processes. Care must be taken, however, not to encumber the process by involving too many people and slowing the decision-making process.

Two committees that should be established include an executive committee consisting of senior management and a steering committee consisting primarily of middle management. The executive committee should be the primary decision-making body for all computerization issues. This committee should meet at least quarterly to review and oversee information system activities.

The steering committee provides the driving force behind the selection effort. The primary function of the steering committee is to coordinate hospital resources in support of the long-range plan and to submit recommendations regarding project priorities and budgets to the executive committee. During the selection process, committee members will participate directly in detailed aspects of system evaluation. Ad hoc task forces also should be established on an as-needed basis to assist in the planning, selection, or implementation of specific aspects of the project.

The information systems project manager is the person responsible for keeping the project on schedule and within budget, and for communicating project status to management. Although the information systems department usually has primary responsibility for selecting new systems, the importance of user involvement cannot be overstated. It is the acceptance and use of the new system, not the sophistication of the system, that determines future success. The project manager should solicit user input throughout the process to ensure that key users become as educated in the strengths and weaknesses of the selected system as the information systems team. By assisting in developing selection criteria and evaluating alternative systems, users develop ownership in the decision and work harder to achieve a successful implementation.

Defining System Requirements

Proper and complete definition of the institution's requirements for computer software and hardware is one of the most critical steps in the selection process. The requirements provide the basis against which alternatives will be measured. The appropriate level of detail in defining user requirements varies from selection to selection. Unless system development is being considered as an alternative, an exhaustive level of detail is not needed to adequately evaluate different products.

After defining functional requirements, the institution should prioritize the requirements into at least two groups: essential features and desired features. Essential features/capabilities can either be identified subjectively (by individual departments) or more objectively (based on benefits to be obtained, such as cost savings, cost avoidance, or increased revenue).

Additional requirements to be identified for the new system include:

- Central processing unit and peripheral hardware
- Critical data elements
- Predefined and ad hoc reporting
- System and data security
- System interfaces
- Other technical capabilities

With system requirements fully identified and prioritized, the institution can proceed with comparative vendor analysis.

Techniques for Evaluating Vendors

Various techniques are available for evaluating vendor systems. Each provides a differing degree of information, and depending on the specific needs of the institution, various techniques may be used together to obtain a complete comparative analysis of the vendor products. A great deal of information about the systems can come from the vendors' marketing representatives, but no institution should rely solely upon these representatives for complete information. Evaluation techniques include:

- *Published comparisons.* Several organizations publish vendor directories and system evaluations. These comparisons provide some useful statistics about the vendors and information about general system capabilities. They provide an excellent starting point for first-time buyers. Comparisons of this type can be quite useful for assisting organizations in identifying software package candidates.
- *Request for information (RFI).* An RFI is a document used to obtain detailed descriptions about individual vendor systems. The RFI generally

is used when relatively little information is known about vendors and information is desired from approximately 10 to 15 different vendors. The RFI is used to solicit general information about the vendor, application system, hardware supported, client information, and general cost so that a subset of vendors can be identified to receive the request for proposal.

- *Consultant reviews.* Consultants knowledgeable in the state of the art in ambulatory care systems would be able to eliminate the need for an RFI by recommending the top five to seven vendors for the institution to evaluate. Consultants provide not only general information about each of the vendors under consideration, but also substantive critiques based on findings from other institutions having selected and implemented various systems. Several consulting firms also sponsor seminars that present strengths and weaknesses of different systems.
- *Presentations.* Presentations are a good way of learning how a software package works and which of its features and capabilities a vendor considers most important. They are particularly useful in updating senior management on the general capabilities of a particular system and vendor in a short period of time. Multiple presentations to different audiences may be necessary to learn about different functional and technical factors related to the system.
- *Request for proposal (RFP).* The RFP provides a very effective approach for comparing candidate systems to the requirements of the health care institution. It provides a formal framework in which the vendor must respond to a set of established requirements. Depending on the magnitude of these requirements, the vendor's response may require from four to five weeks to complete.

    The RFP serves not only as a useful tool for comparative analysis, but also for recording vendor contract commitments. The RFP should include:
    - A description of the organization and business environment
    - A description of the information systems department and current computer systems
    - Special instructions and conditions of proposing
    - Inquiries about the vendor organization, corporate structure, financial status, development history, client base, and user groups
    - Functional requirements for each of the application areas under consideration
    - Technical requirements including environment considerations, response time guarantees, redundancy, hardware, operating systems, interfaces, data security, maintenance, and warranties
    - A request for the recommended vendor-supported training programs and technical/user documentation
    - A request for both one-time and recurring costs.
- *Proposal evaluation.* Various methodologies are available for evaluating proposal results. The two most popular methodologies are the numer-

ical analysis and the ranking analysis. The numerical analysis consists of assigning a weight of 1 to 3 to each requirement based on importance (figure 6-1). Vendor responses are also assigned a numerical value, depending on whether the capabilities are identified as installed and operational, demonstrable, in development, or not planned. The priority value of these requirements and the vendor ratings are multiplied and summed for each application and for the proposal as a whole. Each vendor's score is divided by the total possible score to develop percentages for each application and for the entire proposal. These percentages can then be compared to proposed system costs to obtain a dollar value for the functionality provided.

A primary drawback to this technique is the inability to properly identify numerical scales. It is very easy to skew results to one group of vendors or another based on the numerical scales selected. A vendor's scores should not be viewed as an absolute indication of the vendor's capability to meet the organization's requirements. To minimize bias introduced into the analysis with the numerical ratings, the numerical results should be used to determine vendor groupings, with the highest group receiving further evaluation and other vendors dropped from further consideration.

The ranking technique assigns a value of one through n for each of the n vendors under consideration based on a subjective review of the vendor responses. Although easier to apply, this technique does not fairly reflect the closeness of vendors who are very comparable in satisfying a particular need. A provision should exist in which vendors that equally satisfy a particular set of features receive an equal ranking; those that are comparable should receive a similarly close ranking.

Because a truly objective analysis is impossible, the ideal evaluation methodology is one that is flexible and easy to apply and takes into account subtle differences among vendors.

Figure 6-1.   Example of Numerical Analysis for Proposal Evaluation

Application DD				
Requirement	Assigned Weight	Vendor A Response	Response Value	Weighted Value
1. Duplicate order checking	3	Operational	4	12
2. Transaction logs	1	Development	2	2
3. Renew recurring orders	2	Demonstrable	3	6
4. Help screens	2	Not planned	1	2
	8			22

Total possible value = 8 × 4 = 32
Vendor A total value = 22
Percentage Vendor A = 69%

Note: Weights and values shown are for illustration only. Values will vary for each institution.

- *Demonstrations.* Vendor demonstrations are a useful way to validate proposal responses and to evaluate how effectively the system would perform in the user's environment. Most vendor demonstrations are designed to showcase ease of use of specific capabilities, but generally do not display the system's full capabilities. Demonstration schedules should allow adequate time to permit each demonstration group to ask specific questions and direct the demonstration along the lines the group is most interested in seeing. Although the demonstration may proceed less smoothly, the end result will be a much more fully evaluated system. Emphasis also should be placed on viewing the system's capability to be modified and adapted to the user's needs.

- *Telephone reference checks.* The most reliable information about a particular system comes from current users of the system. Reference checks and site visits provide the best means of evaluating how well the vendor products actually perform in a live environment. The time should be taken to contact various users at several different client sites for each vendor under final consideration.

   Major factors that should be determined from reference checks are the vendor's ability to meet schedules, provide required maintenance, and support the system. Care should be taken to obtain both technical facts and opinions.

- *Site visits.* One of the last but most important steps in the evaluation of systems is viewing the system in total operation in one or more client sites. This is the only way to truly evaluate how well the system performs in an operational environment and how it can be applied to the prospective buyer's environment. Care should be taken to visit sites using the latest release of the system being considered. The visitor also should be wary of facilities that have heavily modified the vendor's software and, therefore, demonstrate more functionality than would actually be obtained from the vendor. Emphasis during site visits should be placed on evaluating the system's effectiveness, vendor performance, user acceptance, problems and mistakes, management and organizational issues, adequacy of computer hardware, adequacy of vendor training and documentation, and overall success or failure. Problems should be discussed openly with the facility and vendor to determine the specific cause.

- *Benchmark tests.* With computer hardware constantly evolving, it is not always possible to visit a facility using the same hardware and software as that proposed by a prospective vendor. In these instances, the prospective buyer should ensure that the vendor conducts benchmark tests on the hardware being proposed. Benchmark testing assesses the feasibility of the proposed hardware and software serving your automation needs: it is a litmus test for information systems. Attending the benchmark test is not necessary, but the prospective buyer should review the results of the benchmark and have the full test explained. Because a benchmark cannot approximate the complexity of the live production environment, relying upon such results is risky. Occasionally, however, it is a risk that must be taken.

- *Corporate visits.* Before selecting a particular system to install, it is important for the prospective buyer to fully understand the philosophy and corporate structure of the company with whom the buyer will be doing business. A visit should be made to the corporate office of each finalist to meet with the company's senior management and to evaluate the support organization, development plans, size of the development group, financial statements, and size of the organization. Only by making such a visit to corporate headquarters and meeting with company management can the prospective buyer learn the true character of the company and gain the confidence needed to enter into a long-term relationship.

Planning and Organizing for Implementation

After system selection and contract negotiations are concluded, the institution is ready to begin the task of implementation. Much of the planning should have been completed during the contracting process. Major milestones and resource requirements associated with the implementation should be included in the contract. All software enhancements that the vendor will be making specifically for the buying institution, and all interfaces required to connect other institutions' systems, should also be specified in the contract.

Before selecting an implementation strategy, there are several issues that the institution should analyze:

- Is the current information systems staff adequate to continue maintenance on current systems as well as implement the new system?
- Does the information systems staff possess the proper mix of technical and user-oriented knowledge to implement the new system?
- Does the institution have the necessary project management experience to properly manage and control the implementation?
- How much training is required to get the institution's staff completely oriented to the new system?
- How much modification to the delivered system is required to meet the institution's needs?
- How much ongoing maintenance to the system will be required?
- What implementation approaches does the software vendor support and recommend?

On the basis of answers to these questions and others specific to each institution, the institution should select an implementation strategy.

(A more detailed treatment of implementation options is discussed in chapter 5.) One possible strategy is for the institution to implement the entire system independent of the vendor. This should be considered only if the institution has a strong information systems staff, an experienced project manager, and heavy user involvement.

Another alternative is for the vendor to install the system. Although it may be costly, this alternative can work well for turnkey installations and for institutions with little in-house staff. Because little working knowledge of the system is acquired by institution staff, the institution remains heavily dependent upon the vendor for all support and future modifications.

The most widely accepted alternative is shared responsibility between institution and vendor. This alternative provides the institution with the working knowledge necessary for making minor system enhancements and modifications and yet minimizes ongoing staff requirements. The vendor or a third-party consultant can provide such services as analyst support, project management, user training, hardware and facilities planning, software modification, interface development, conversion assistance, procedure development, and implementation audits.

Regardless of the strategy selected, there are several steps that the institution should take to organize its internal efforts. As in the selection process, users should be heavily involved and play an active role in the implementation. Although other department commitments are heavy, and departments/clinics are often tightly staffed, adequate time must be dedicated to support the implementation. In addition to a primary project team identified by the institution, committees and user liaisons from various departments and clinics should be established.

A project manager should be designated and analysts/programmers assigned to the project team as required. Also represented in the project should be technical support, vendor support, an education coordinator, and a benefits/quality assurance specialist. Technical support will handle all the site preparation, hardware, system software, and telecommunications issues. If a single individual cannot be designated as education coordinator to handle the preparation of training guides for user training, the implementation analysts will have to perform this function. The benefits/quality assurance specialist is responsible for streamlining system use, expediting policy and procedure changes, auditing testing and training, and maximizing benefits derived from system use.

In addition to the primary project team, user liaisons from the various departments and clinics should be identified. These individuals will work with the implementation analysts in defining modifications to the system and in training system users. The executive committee and steering committee established during the selection process should continue to meet throughout the implementation to monitor progress, resolve issues, revise policies, and ensure coordination throughout the institution. Specific task forces may be established to concentrate on implementation activities or issues during the project.

Because of the large number of implementation tasks that must be planned and scheduled before an implementation can begin, ample time should be allowed for developing and communicating the plan throughout the institution. With the resources identified, the next step is to develop a detailed work plan by defining the individual project tasks and estimating the number of workdays by skill level required to complete each task.

Implementation Activities

With the implementation and resource plan completed, actual implementation activities can begin. These activities will vary from institution to institution, depending upon the approach selected and the system being implemented. Specific tasks that are likely to be required are presented below:

- *Recruit personnel.* Having identified the resources required to implement and support the system, recruitment of needed personnel should begin. The institution should determine the number of personnel required on an ongoing basis and consider contracting for supplemental personnel or personnel with specialized skills. Inside candidates should be given first consideration because of their operational knowledge and contacts. Technical positions (for example, programmers or computer operators) would probably be filled from the outside unless a service bureau or facilities management arrangement has been established.
- *Prepare the computer room.* This task involves preparing a new site or updating a current computer room site to provide adequate space, power, fire prevention, safety, lighting, security, and environmental conditions.
- *Install communication lines.* Considering the terminal and printer deployment locations throughout the institution, cable must be installed to all locations. If the system will be supporting users in multiple buildings, communication lines or microwave transmitters/receivers must be installed in each building.
- *Install hardware.* This task involves unpacking, executing diagnostics, and installing system hardware. Central processing unit hardware and peripherals are usually installed by the hardware vendor. Terminal and printer installation may be handled by institution personnel.
- *Train the project team.* Implementation analysts, project management, and technical support personnel should attend vendor-sponsored

classes. These classes may be held at the vendor's training facility at the installation site, depending on the number of people attending, course logistics, and type of personnel being trained. Many vendors prefer to have the majority of training provided offsite for implementation personnel and onsite for operations personnel.

- *Collect data.* During this task, institution-specific facts, policies, and procedures are gathered from each department and clinic. The information obtained is analyzed, and specifications for design and use of the system within the department/clinic are prepared. All changes to screens and reports are identified during this task.
- *Order supplies.* All necessary forms, paper, printer ribbons, and spare equipment parts should be ordered and stored onsite.
- *Do system coding/modification.* This task involves making changes to screens, reports, forms, and parameter tables as defined in the specifications developed during the data collection task. Any specialized software development to be completed by the institution or the vendor is also completed during this period.
- *Do interface and conversion coding.* This task involves defining detailed specifications and writing the necessary software routines to interface appropriate systems and convert current data files to the new system. This task needs to begin early in the implementation process to allow adequate time for unforeseen delays, particularly if a number of different vendors are involved.
- *Do procedure documentation.* This task involves modifying institutional/departmental policies and procedures as appropriate to maximize efficient use of the new system. Technical documentation for computer operations and technical support should also be developed or updated as needed. Manual backup procedures to be used when the system is down should be developed for all affected departments.
- *Perform system testing.* Each function of the system must be tested to demonstrate that it conforms to the specifications identified during the data collection period. After required corrections have been made, users should formally sign off that specifications have been met. After this functional testing, integrated systems testing should be conducted. Various patient scenarios should be run through the system to verify that the system functions properly on an institutionwide basis. When the integrated test is completed successfully, the system is ready for activation.
- *Conduct user training.* Depending on the education plan developed at the beginning of the project, either the education coordinator or the user departments should prepare training guides to correspond with the modified system. Although some training can be done in individual departments, it may be necessary to set up a training room for training large groups of personnel. Consideration should be given to setting up a training methodology that not only supports the implementation but

also will continue the training of future new employees as normal turnover occurs in the organization. Computer-based training offers significant advantages over traditional training methods for both initial and ongoing education.

The implementation analysts or education coordinator can either personally train all institution personnel or can train designated trainers in each department/clinic. Many vendors and consultants believe that departmental staff should train their own employees because they are more knowledgeable about individual personalities and can better determine the amount of training required for each employee. Proficiency tests should be administered before user access codes are assigned. The institution may wish to consider having the employees sign nondisclosure statements at the time access codes are issued.

- *Perform system activation.* When testing and training are completed, files should be converted and live patient data should be loaded into the system. If a current system is being replaced, the institution may choose to run the new system in tandem for a specified period of time until confidence is gained in the new system.

  If an old system is being converted, the institution may be forced to convert the entire system at one time. If the institution is converting from a manual operation, a phased implementation may be preferred. With a phased implementation, information systems analysts could concentrate on one user group at a time and, therefore, better control the conversion.

- *Conduct postimplementation review.* After users have become comfortable with use of the system (generally three to six months after activation), a postimplementation review of the system should be conducted. This review should include system design, documentation, adequacy of hardware, procedure compliance, and user satisfaction. The person conducting the audit should verify whether original objectives established by the project team and by each department/clinic have been realized. The auditor should also verify that any benefits originally expected from the system have, in fact, been realized. If benefits have not been realized, the auditor should determine the reasons why and recommend corrective action.

Conclusion

Various strategies and methodologies have been presented for evaluating, selecting, and implementing ambulatory information systems. Different strategies will be appropriate based upon the specific needs, experience, resources, and constraints of the buying institution. Each institution must determine for itself which approach can best accomplish system objectives.

No matter what strategy or set of strategies are followed for selecting and implementing new ambulatory systems, there are several factors that can greatly affect project success and should be emphasized by each institution:

- Heavy senior management involvement and commitment
- Comprehensive long-range information systems plan
- Realistic user expectations
- Extensive user involvement
- Adequate departmental support
- Comprehensive user education
- Positive user attitudes
- Proper allocation of resources
- Physician commitment
- Strong project control and management
- Timely resolution of issues
- Adequate hardware configuration
- Software and hardware reliability
- Flexibility to adapt to changing needs

If appropriate attention is given to each of these factors, most of the common mistakes and performance deficiencies can be avoided.

Chapter 7

Achieving Information Systems Benefits

O. John Kralovec

Almost anyone working with information systems has had an opportunity to go through a cost-justification process at one time or another. Identifying potential benefits from a new information system is not a new trend. However, what we are experiencing in today's health care environment is a renewed focus on determining the extent of potential benefits and a significant emphasis on ensuring that computer benefits are actually achieved. Over the years, many organizations have purchased and installed information systems with the expectation that significant benefits would accrue. Often it was found that once the systems were installed, benefits were not realized, anticipated savings never materialized, and some system-related expenditures actually increased. Achieving benefits from information systems has become not only an economic necessity but, for many institutions, will mean the difference between success or failure in the future.

In the context of this chapter, *benefits* are the advantages derived from effective installation and operation of computer systems. Benefits address the tangible impact systems have upon an organization. *Benefit realization* is the process by which hospital management mobilizes and commits resources to realize the potential benefits from information systems.

Current Trends

There are five major forces behind the renewed emphasis and focus on benefit realization:

- Increased need to cost-justify systems
- Increased focus on benefits by system vendors

- Need for improved operational control
- Focus on enhanced quality
- Hospital participation in the identification and achievement of benefits

As costs for information systems continue to increase, and as the expenditures for systems continue to use more resources, hospital management is increasingly concerned that these systems be cost-justified. Boards of directors are becoming more critical in evaluating system purchases, and senior health care executives are being held increasingly accountable for demonstrating a tangible financial return on the investment in systems. In addition, we see the cost-justification process not only extending to new systems but to replacement systems and enhancements of current systems as well. Detailed cost justification has become an essential part of the entire system selection decision-making process, and this trend will continue.

Another key trend is the focus on benefit identification and realization by information systems vendors as a means of differentiating their various products in the crowded marketplace. Some of the most successful vendors today are the ones that have made a significant commitment not only to ensure that their systems provide tangible benefits for their clients, but to develop a methodology so that hospitals realize these benefits. As the systems decisions to be made by hospital managers and executives become more complex, this focus by information systems vendors on benefit identification and realization will become increasingly important to successful competition in the information systems arena. Information systems' functional capabilities, flexibility, ease of use, *and* benefit potential are all being stressed by information systems vendors to support this benefit orientation.

As hospitals struggle to maintain profitability and respond to the dramatic changes that are occurring in the industry, information systems are expected to provide for improved operational control. Systems in the future must be responsive to supporting optimal operating methods and procedures in the workplace, thereby enhancing levels of productivity, quality, and service. In addition, as organizations are going through restructuring, it is critical for information systems to be responsive to the changing roles of both managers and employees. They must also carry out requirements for a flexible and dynamic approach to staffing and organizing departmental operations. The ability of information systems to provide benefits that will result in improved clinical practice is another trend that is beginning and probably will continue in the future. Another key area related to the benefits from installing information systems is the potential impact on recruitment and retention, particularly in nursing areas. The information systems vendors who will be most successful in the future are the ones that demonstrate they can assist hospitals in optimizing productivity levels, streamlining day-to-day operations, and enhancing quality of service.

Quality is becoming an increasingly important aspect of service delivery in the health care industry. For many institutions, level of quality will become the primary market differentiator and the key to protecting and expanding their market share. Although there has not been a significant focus on quality in the past, this is rapidly changing, and in the future we will see extensive efforts oriented toward defining and monitoring quality and ensuring that quality standards are maintained. Information systems will play a significant and vital role in quality enhancement and will be a major contributor to efforts to improve quality and service. Purchases of systems that do not provide tangible benefits in these areas will have a difficult time being justified by hospital management.

An important factor neglected in the past that is now recognized as critical to the success of benefit realization is involving hospital managers and employees in the identification and achievement of information systems benefits. A more traditional approach has been for the management information systems department, hospital administration, outside consultants, or vendors to provide the focus for a benefit identification process. Given the complexity of the information systems currently available in the industry and their impact on operations, and given the importance of employee buy-in and participation in the process, it is absolutely essential to have a participative benefit approach involving almost everyone affected by the new information system. This means that key users are involved in (1) looking at how information systems will affect their departments, (2) determining the expected level of benefits, and (3) developing the methodologies and implementation strategy to make sure that information systems benefits are achieved. In our experience, this process results in a more realistic assessment of the probable impact of information systems on hospital operations. In addition, it is the only way to ensure high levels of commitment to identified potential benefits and active involvement in making sure that these benefits are actually achieved once information systems have been installed.

Benefit Realization Opportunities

The benefit process can be examined in two distinct phases: identification and development/implementation of a plan to make sure that changes identified (in methods, procedures, staffing, and so forth) are actually implemented and tangible outcomes are realized. When looking at the whole process of benefit realization, it is important to acknowledge that opportunities for improvement exist in most operating environments. There are usually ways to improve work flow and task assignment, as well as enhance work distribution and productivity levels.

Changes in these areas can result in enhanced quality of service or reduced staffing requirements. An information system is another tool for improving the way things are done operationally and managerially in any given health care area. A focused and aggressive management engineering approach in a particular operational area will undoubtedly provide significant benefits; installing an information system also has potential for providing benefits. However, the combination of the two yields the greatest overall benefit and ensures that the role of information systems in enhancing departmental operations is fully realized.

The vendors in the marketplace who have been the most successful in demonstrating tangible benefits from information systems have also focused on improving and streamlining operations through traditional management engineering techniques. In many cases, the tremendous benefits that have been identified and realized by hospital executives result as much from operational methods improvements as from installing information systems. Therefore, it is important to realize that an institution's willingness to commit resources to a detailed evaluation of operational performance in a particular area directly affects the level of benefits realized from a computer system in that area. In many cases, it is the operational improvements rather than the information system per se that yield the most substantial benefits to the organization. Identifying operational enhancements and then structuring information systems to support optimal operations yields the greatest overall benefit.

Ideally, the benefit realization process should begin with an assessment of current departmental operations, methods and procedures, work flow, skill mix, task assignment, and organizational structure. These factors should be carefully evaluated, opportunities for improvement should be identified, and a new performance model should be developed that optimizes these factors. Information systems should be evaluated in terms of how they can support optimum departmental operations and what degree of system customization or enhancements are required. This ensures that information systems support high levels of productivity and quality of service, rather than having departmental operations organized to support an information system. Hospitals that are either unwilling or unable to commit the resources to this process will never fully realize the total potential benefit from improvements in these critical areas.

If hospitals are unable to perform this type of assessment and evaluation before information systems are actually installed, it is important to begin to address these issues during the process of defining systems-related procedures and preimplementation activities. As hospital representatives, users, and key departmental personnel are evaluating information systems, looking at new procedures resulting from information systems, and determining the impact of systems on their operations, questions should be raised concerning the optimal way of doing things in the department. This focus will result in challenging old ways of doing things and long-standing assumptions about how the work should be performed. This perspective will result in a more efficient use of resources in any given area. It is important to realize that in many cases, information systems were not designed to optimize overall department work flow, methods, and procedures. Often system design decisions are made without looking at the departmental operating environment; therefore, many of the interactions and coordinations of various functions may have been neglected.

Anyone who has gone through a system conversion has realized that this process provides a unique opportunity for hospitals to reevaluate long-standing policy, procedural, and operational issues. It is imperative to take advantage of this process and ensure that the time and effort spent by hospital personnel to prepare for and install information systems be used to its fullest. The unique opportunity this process affords to thoroughly evaluate how things are being done and identify innovative, creative solutions to operational problems should not be missed. It is imperative that hospitals use this opportunity to make changes, identify new methods and procedures, and work with department managers to ensure that operations will support the goals and objectives of the institution.

Types of Benefits

There are four basic categories of systems-related benefits. They include:

- *Fiscal management:* The ability to ensure the financial viability of the institution, including asset protection, optimization of cash flow, and maintaining appropriate debt-to-capital ratios.
- *Clinical management:* The ability to provide appropriate patient care services that maximize the utilization of resources and result in appropriate outcomes.
- *Human resource management:* The ability to recruit, train, and maintain an appropriate work force that can deliver both services and products in an efficient manner.
- *Image management:* The ability to successfully implement programs and services that enhance the external perceptions of the facility by physicians, patients, volunteers, and the community at large.

Fiscal Management

A significant opportunity exists for information systems to provide fiscal management benefits. Often the most significant benefits realized from a computer system will be in the areas of accounts receivable, cash flow, and inventory management. Enhancing billing and collection functions,

increasing cash flow, and reducing inventories are all areas where computer systems will provide significant benefits to an organization. In addition, information systems can be extremely valuable in identifying
opportunities to reduce overall operating expenses and then providing
the mechanisms to monitor the achievement of goals in these key areas.
Fiscal management is an increasingly important function of information
systems support and one that needs to be addressed very carefully in
the benefit identification process. Typical fiscal management benefits of
systems implementation include the following:

- Reduced days in accounts receivable
- Increased cash flow
- Reduced inventories
- Enhanced revenues
- Reduced operating expenses
- Improved collection of patient information
- Improved quality/breadth of financial information
- Better forecasting for capital, operations, and expense budgeting
- Improved tracking of vendor information and avoidance of duplicate
  payments
- Improved ability to allocate costs

Clinical Management

While hospitals are putting emphasis on controlling operating expenses,
clinical management is also becoming an increasingly important area for
most health care institutions. There is a greater focus on quality improvement and the use of information systems to assist in improving accuracy,
increasing timeliness, and enhancing overall service levels. Information
systems designed to support nursing practice (for example, care planning, charting, and documentation) are becoming more readily available
and are beginning to demonstrate tangible benefits. These trends will
continue; identified clinical management benefits will become a significant reason for justifying information systems. Typical clinical management benefits include:

- Improved quality and timeliness of clinical and demographic infor-
  mation
- Improved patient processing and flow
- Enhanced scope of information captured
- Improved patient monitoring
- Increased accuracy in determining components of a patient stay or visit
- Enhanced accuracy of nursing and ancillary documentation
- Increased time available for direct patient care
- Increased availability of medical data for clinical decision making

Human Resource Management

One of the primary areas of benefits traditionally identified has been potential savings in full-time equivalents (FTEs). Reducing staffing levels has been a key consideration in selecting information systems. Although this will continue to be a focus for information systems, in the future the emphasis will shift toward broader human resource management issues. Information systems have the ability to support improved management of staff skill mix in various departmental areas, improved resource utilization, and improved recruitment and retention efforts. Department managers and administration are much more willing to support information systems when the benefits are seen in a broader human resource management context and not just in terms of reducing staff. System benefits directly affecting the utilization and management of human resources include:

- Reduction in FTEs
- Reduction in payroll expenses due to changes in skill mix
- Ability to attract and hire new employees with appropriate skills
- Reduction in turnover
- Improved employee satisfaction
- Improved employee utilization
- Ability to monitor productivity and conduct work-load analyses
- Avoidance of growth in staff to deal with additional tasks

Image Management

Community perceptions of the effectiveness of an institution are becoming increasingly important to an institution's success in a particular marketplace. Information systems are playing a more important role in enhancing the image of institutions—not only in the community but also with the medical staff and other key constituencies. Improving information systems support to the medical staff not only provides immediate tangible benefits in terms of assisting with the practice of medicine, but it is also an important means of building relationships that will strengthen physician ties to the institutions. Information systems will become more important in helping an institution define its position in the industry and communicate its commitment to state-of-the-art technologies to ensure optimal patient care. It is not uncommon for institutions today to identify image and image management as key differentiators of their services, and computer systems will continue to provide a significant advantage in this area. In addition, it is becoming clear that information systems will be of great help in assisting an institution in maintaining its strategic competitive advantage; in some cases, information systems will mean the difference between dominating a particular market and struggling to survive. Examples of image management benefits include:

- Enhanced medical staff relations and communications
- Improved public image
- Ability to maintain or increase physician referrals or facilitation of joint ventures with physicians and other health care groups
- Ability to maintain or improve the institution's competitive position in the marketplace
- Improved ability to monitor donations and endowments
- Improved ability to identify external referral sources

Quantitative and Qualitative Benefits

In looking at the benefit realization process, it is important to recognize that different types of benefits will be achieved through the installation of an information system. Some will be easier to identify and measure than others, but a wide variety and scope of benefits are possible. *Quantitative benefits* are those benefits to which dollar amounts can be assigned. They are measurable, and their achievement can be evaluated after system implementation. Examples of quantitative benefits include:

- FTE reductions
- Savings in forms and supplies
- Reductions in inventories
- Reductions in days in accounts receivable

Qualitative benefits are those benefits to which specific dollar amounts cannot be easily assigned. Improvement in employee morale, for example, is a qualitative but intangible benefit of automation. Employees may learn new job skills, gain greater satisfaction, and even experience career advancement as a result of automation. These results, however, are difficult to measure in terms of how many dollars are saved. Other examples of qualitative benefits include:

- Improved public image
- Improved quality of information
- Improved medical staff communications

Qualitative benefits, while not usually assigned dollar values, can still be measured, however. The utilization of opinion surveys, turnover analysis, physician referral analysis, and so forth, can serve to measure qualitative benefits before and after system implementation.

Many benefit realization projects have failed to achieve their desired result simply because hospital employees and managers did not "buy in" to benefits identified for the particular system. It is essential for employees to believe that the process of identifying benefits has addressed the total scope of potential opportunities (both quantitative and qualitative) and that a balanced and equitable view has been taken in relation to potential opportunity. Employees are willing to support a benefit realization process if they understand the nature of the benefits identified and if they believe that the potential impact of the system has been thoroughly evaluated. During the identification of benefits, managers are increasingly hesitant to commit only to those benefits that will result in potential reductions in staff. A more acceptable approach, and one that generates greater employee support, is a comprehensive and balanced one that addresses both quantitative and qualitative benefits in the areas of fiscal, clinical, human resource, and image management.

Benefit Realization Methodology

Hospital commitment to a benefit realization methodology ensures that managers and other key personnel are actually able to realize the benefits anticipated from implementing a new information system. It is critical to the success of this process that the following assumptions become part of the overall institutional philosophy regarding benefit realization:

- Recognize that benefits achievement is an institutional expectation.
- Get department managers to commit to a work plan that specifies tasks/activities, responsibilities, and due dates for benefit realization activities.
- Use acceptable measures and quantification tools to assess benefits and achievements.
- Implement a monitoring system to track progress toward plan objectives at specific time intervals.

Once hospital administrators, managers, and key employees understand and support these assumptions, the benefit realization process continues with the following steps:

1. Confirmation of benefit goals and objectives
2. Development of a benefit action plan (work plan)
3. Collection of baseline data
4. Evaluation of progress

Confirmation of Benefit Goals and Objectives

The key to ensuring support for the achievement of information systems benefits lies in the process that is used to identify potential benefits and then determine the appropriate benefit goals and objectives. All department managers and key personnel affected by information systems must be a part of this process and must participate fully in the benefit identification and planning process. This ensures that managers and other key employees have confidence that the benefits identified can actually be achieved. When hospital personnel are directly involved in the process of identifying benefits and establishing benefit goals and objectives, they are much more willing to commit to improving performance levels based on information systems implementation. There are four steps in this process that are critical for employee participation, involvement, and buy-in:

• Identification of potential benefits
• Determination of qualitative and quantitative benefits
• Assessment of benefit areas
• Identification of benefit savings and impact

Benefit identification begins by looking at the current departmental operating environment, identifying current methods and procedures (how people are really doing things), and then determining specific changes resulting from the new information system. Key hospital personnel in each functional area must document current departmental operations and review, in detail, new procedures associated with the new information system to determine how their current methods and procedures will change. Involving hospital personnel at all levels in this process provides an opportunity to identify operational improvement opportunities, reevaluate methods and procedures, and assess areas where enhancements can be made. This not only increases understanding of the current operating environment, but it also results in improved understanding of the operating environment with the new information system. By going through this process and anticipating changes, employees are better able to identify benefits that will occur as a result of the new system.

Taking a comprehensive approach to quantitative and qualitative benefits is essential to the success of this type of effort. A focus on both types of benefits will lead to greater employee buy-in and a higher degree of success overall. The natural inclination is for managers to highlight qualitative and less tangible benefits and to place lesser emphasis on quantitative benefits that will result in FTE reductions or other hard-dollar savings. If tangible, bottom-line savings are a requirement for installing a system, this must be made a high priority for hospital personnel. Qualitative benefits can still be identified and evaluated, but anticipated outcomes and operational, organizational, or other behavioral changes must be clearly identified, measured, and evaluated after implementation. The process of quantifying benefits in some areas may be difficult for hospital managers and other affected personnel; however, the process ensures a better understanding of the potential impact of information systems and provides a vehicle to make sure that changes are actually realized.

Most hospital strategic plans address clinical, fiscal, human resource, and image management areas. Information systems should facilitate the attainment of key strategic goals and objectives and support operational methods that are consistent with the mission of the institution. A major problem with developing goals and objectives in institutions typically has been the lack of consistency between strategic goals and objectives and individual departmental goals and objectives. Information systems benefits and specific departmental goals and objectives for achieving those benefits should be evaluated in light of the overall strategy and direction of the institution. Developing goals and objectives should not be a bottom-up process of identifying departmental benefit areas, but should start with the key success factors identified for the institution as a whole and then work backward to determine the exact impact on each specific departmental area. It is important to ensure that the benefit areas determined at a departmental level are consistent with the priorities of the institution overall, and that information systems will be affecting the operational areas essential to support the long-range goals of the institution.

Determining estimated savings is a critical component of the benefit achievement process. Savings in terms of forms reductions, supply/inventory reductions, and other cost-avoidance measures are relatively straightforward and easy to determine. It is important not to distort potential cost savings by aggregating increments of time that will be saved randomly throughout the day by various employees (for example, .5 FTE plus .2 FTE plus .3 FTE does not necessarily equal 1.0 FTE). Savings in FTEs must be realistic and must be consistent with the operating requirements and demands of each departmental area. A useful distinction can be made between savings that are theoretically "available" and savings that are actually "achievable." Another benefit (and potential opportunity) lies in the area of cost avoidance: those situations where an institution will avoid adding staff, acquiring additional resources, or increasing expenditures as a result of specific applications of the information systems. Estimating savings is a critical part of the entire process and one that needs very careful attention and thorough review and evaluation by all employees affected in the institution.

Development of a Benefit Action Plan

The action plan, essential to a successful benefit realization effort, is the blueprint that department managers and key personnel will use in achieving the benefits identified for information systems in their particular areas (figure 7-1). The plan not only summarizes the key activities

Figure 7-1. Benefit Action Plan

Facility: _____

Admin./VP: _____

Department: _____

Cost center: _____

Prepared by: _____   Title: Manager

Approved by: _____   Title: Director

Date: _____

page __1__ of __1__

Objective Number	Major Area	Objective/Task/Activity Description	Start mo/day/yr	Stop mo/day/yr	Responsibility Primary	Secondary
01.00.00	Human resources	Determine time saved in locating films	11-1-87	4-30-88	Clerk	Assistant
02.00.00	Image	Assess communications with other departments	4-1-88	Ongoing	Assistant	Manager
03.00.00	Clinical	Assess timeliness in providing patient information	4-1-88	4-30-88	Assistant	Manager
04.00.00	Clinical	Evaluate the utilization of equipment	4-1-88	4-30-88	Assistant	Manager
05.00.00	Human resources	Determine savings in producing film jackets	4-1-88	4-30-88	Clerk	Assistant
06.00.00	Image	Document improvement in patient scheduling	4-1-88	4-30-88	Manager	
07.00.00	Fiscal	Validate improved charge capture	5-1-88	5-5-88	Manager	Finance Department
08.00.00	Human resources	Validate increased productivity	5-1-88	5-5-88	Manager	Human Resources Department
09.00.00	VALUE	Complete VALUE Analysis Report	5-6-88	5-15-88	Manager	

that need to be performed, along with individual responsibilities, but it also provides the vehicle for tracking progress, evaluating milestones, and determining the overall effectiveness of benefit achievement efforts to date. The development of the action plan is actually one of the more difficult parts of the process simply because this is an activity that most department managers are not used to performing. Although it will undoubtedly take some time to develop and refine an action plan, the process is absolutely essential to ensure that department managers and other key personnel have the tools necessary to successfully manage benefit realization efforts. It also provides the foundation for the step-by-step attainment of operational improvements and savings.

Benefit action plans need to clearly and thoroughly identify each area that will be affected by information systems and the benefits (clinical, human resources, fiscal, and image) associated with each one of those areas. For each area, precise action steps need to be developed that clearly specify all of the activities necessary to accomplish the achievement of benefits. It is important that all the activities be carefully delineated and that the action plan has been developed in enough detail to ensure that each step is identified and can be successfully executed.

It is strongly recommended that benefit objectives be built into the hospital's overall performance appraisal system and that managers be held accountable for accomplishing benefit objectives just as they would personal, professional, or operational objectives normally developed during the course of the year. Building benefit objectives into the performance appraisal process will provide an important link between implementing systems and providing incentives and opportunities for recognition of managers related to benefit achievement.

Collection of Baseline Data

Proper measurement is essential in evaluating benefit accomplishment and in ensuring that benefits are actually achieved. Preimplementation data gathering should occur approximately two to four months before system installation. This will allow enough of a trend to be established so that an effective baseline can be developed and postimplementation measurement can more accurately represent the actual degree of benefit achievement. This provides a large enough sampling for effective evaluation with a minimum amount of disruption. It is important that appropriate measures be developed for any benefit areas that have been identified and that an effective baseline be established prior to system implementation. Without an adequate baseline established prior to the start of the process, it will be impossible to correctly or appropriately identify the extent of benefits actually accomplished as a result of the implementation. It is important to identify measures and develop baseline data not only for those areas that can be easily quantified in terms of financial impact but also those areas that relate to quality, service levels, and other "softer" benefits.

Development of measures for benefit areas is a process that should involve hospital executives, administrators, department heads, supervisors, and other key employees affected by the new system. In some cases the measures will be obvious and easy to identify; other cases will require some discussion and creativity to identify the best way to actually measure the expected benefits. The best measures are those where information is easily available, such as payroll statistics, current units of service statistics, current inventory statistics, cost statistics, ratios, and other hospital-generated data. If at all possible, department heads should avoid benefit measures that will require extensive amounts of data collection, work sampling, or collection of statistics not easily available through existing information systems or other departmental logs and records. In some cases, it may be possible to actually incorporate benefit measures into the installation of the system so that the system assists in the collection of key benefit-related information. Measures generated by internal systems or other existing systems will have more credibility when used as a basis of measurement and documentation of actual results achieved.

Evaluation of Progress

Once the system has been stabilized, the policies and procedures have been implemented, the training has been completed, and any software customization or enhancements have been finalized, it is important to begin collecting postimplementation data. The same indicators and sources of data identified earlier in the process should be used to make sure that consistency is maintained between data gathered for the baseline and data gathered for the postimplementation audit. Analysis of results should be conducted on a regular basis, and department heads, managers, and other key individuals should meet regularly to review progress, identify any obstacles, and evaluate progress toward accomplishing tangible savings and other quantifiable results. Figure 7-2 presents a sample progress report used by managers to report the results of the benefit realization process, evaluate their progress toward achieving benefit goals, identify savings or other quantifiable improvements achieved, and identify any areas that require additional attention. This reporting process helps ensure that the project is going as planned, and it provides a formal approach to reviewing and evaluating the impact of information systems on departmental operations. It also allows managers to evaluate their progress in achieving the goals and objectives identified earlier for the system. Undoubtedly a number of unanticipated factors will affect the achievement of benefits; these should be addressed during the review process. The evaluation of progress

Figure 7-2. Sample Progress Report

Memo: Information Systems Operations Committee   **Re:** Implementation of XYZ Computer System
From: John Jones, Department Manager   **Date:** January 1, 1988

I. Confirmation of Actual System Costs

The XYZ Computer System was installed on October 1, 1987. Final costs were as follows:

	Projected	Actual	Variance
Hardware	$50,000	$55,000	$ 5,000
Software	20,000	29,000	9,000
Other	4,000	8,000	4,000
Totals	$74,000	$92,000	$18,000

II. Anticipated Benefits

Benefits were projected in the following areas:

Type	Amount	Dollars
FTE reductions	4.0	$ 80,000
Forms savings		40,000
Other (supplies)		5,000
Total		$125,000

These projected benefits are annual savings.

III. Actual Benefits Realized

After completing the benefits analysis, the following benefits savings were documented:

Type	Amount	Dollars
FTE reductions	3.0	$ 60,000
Forms savings		40,000
Other (supplies)		4,000
Total		$104,000

IV. Variance Report

Costs of the system were higher than anticipated due to the following:

Description	Dollars
Addition of one terminal	$ 5,000
Increased cost of interface	9,000
Consulting assistance	4,000
Total	$18,000

The variance in anticipated benefits is due to the following factors:

Description	Comments
FTE reductions	System functions did not provide maximum savings on data entry
Forms savings	Required to get 3-part forms for computer print, custom format
Other (supplies)	After much evaluation, it was determined to add upgraded printer ribbons required for computer forms

V. Summary Comments

The overall variances then are:

System costs	$18,000
System benefits	21,000
Total	$39,000

It is anticipated that further reductions in FTEs will be possible over the next 9–12 months, provided the vendor can deliver the software upgrades now anticipated during that time frame. It is expected that this would result in a savings of $20,000 per year.

toward achieving benefits should also include a focus on problem solving and should explore ways to maximize the impact of systems in a supportive and proactive manner.

It is important to begin management of progress toward objectives only after the system has been stabilized and users have an opportunity to learn system functions and features. Depending on the nature of the system application, at least six months should be allotted for the stabilization process prior to actual evaluation of the achievement of any benefits. At this point, time should be allowed for the system to become integrated into departmental operations and to ensure that performance levels are not adversely affected by educational or other training-related issues. In addition, users should have the opportunity to achieve a level of proficiency and competence with the new system that allows benefit attainment to become a source of motivation and encouragement for departmental management and users. The status of the implementation should be carefully monitored to ensure that the anticipated impact on operations will in fact be realized and to provide a preliminary assessment of the ability to achieve system benefits. If at this point it appears that the system will not be able to accomplish initial objectives or satisfy initial expectations, changes or enhancements should be initiated to correct this problem or benefit objectives reviewed and revised if possible.

Measurement Techniques

Specific measurement techniques need to be selected that will ensure the hospital's ability to validate realized benefits after implementation of the system. Examples of the various measurement techniques include, but are not limited to, the following:

- *Payroll analysis:* Calculation of the actual number of FTEs based on the total hours paid for a defined period of time.
- *Units of service analysis:* Statistics compiled on the volume of departmental services utilized combined with payroll data for the same period to obtain the ratios of FTEs per unit of service.
- *Inventory analysis:* Calculation of average materials usage per unit of service for specific supply items.
- *Capital equipment analysis:* Calculation of savings associated with the removal or reduction of equipment or growth avoidance savings.
- *Cost analysis:* Calculation of savings in other operating expenses (not included in FTEs, materials, or physical assets), such as outside services.
- *Ratio analysis:* Reduction in days in accounts receivable or number of days supply in inventory.
- *Revenue analysis:* Measurement of the ability to capture previously lost charges or the ability to process more patients, resulting in additional

services provided. Margin analysis can also be used to calculate the relationship between departmental profit and departmental net revenues.

- *Work sampling:* Determination of the change in the percentage of employee time devoted to major activities due to the installation of information systems.
- *Job content analysis:* Measurement of the amount of employee time spent in selected job activities (repetitive and predictable tasks).
- *Error sampling:* Determination of the frequency of errors in activities performed or in information generated.
- *Patient wait time observation:* Measurement of the average time elapsed between patient arrival and either initiation or completion of services.
- *Timeliness analysis:* Measurement of the average turnaround time for identified reports, orders, or procedures.
- *Scaling:* Use of an opinion survey to assess the quality of information in a report generated by automated systems. Measurement should include an assessment of:
  - Timeliness
  - Accuracy
  - Relevance
  - Clarity
  - Quantity of information

Conclusion

Obviously, benefit realization requires a significant amount of effort on the part of various hospital personnel. The major question that needs to be addressed is "What is in it for me?"—that is, what benefits the manager or his or her departmental supervisors and other users will receive from going through the benefit realization process. The following are among the significant reasons directly affecting managers and other users for committing the time and effort necessary for this process:

- Achieving benefits and tangible cost savings will often help relieve pressures to control costs and allow managers to realize tangible savings without resorting to reducing staff or reducing the scope of services.
- The benefit analysis process will result in identifying various ways to simplify work flow, improve methods and procedures, improve task assignment, and enhance work distribution. This will result in smoother departmental operations, reduction in unproductive and unnecessary activities, and increased ability of the department to provide additional services or enhance the quality of service with existing resources.
- Managers who are able to demonstrate tangible savings and operational improvements from installing computer systems establish credi-

bility with administration. This typically results in greater administration support for future information systems requests and improves a manager's ability to continue to provide automated support for his or her department.

- Achieving benefit objectives demonstrates and enhances a manager's ability to manage and thus provides tangible career-enhancing opportunities. In some cases, hospitals have tied benefit achievement to pay for performance or to incentive compensation systems.
- Benefit realization is becoming a key element of a systems installation and an aspect of the implementation process that will become increasingly important in the future. Department managers who are able to take the initiative in this process not only will be contributing substantially to the success of their organization but will also improve the quality of work life for their employees.

Chapter 8

Implications of Prospective Payment

Theodore A. Matson and Margaret D. Sabin

Changing methods of payment for ambulatory care services will have a lasting impact on the delivery of those services in the hospital setting. Therefore, hospitals need to consider likely changes as they look toward organizing and managing ambulatory care services in the future. This chapter will explain how all these changes affect ambulatory care data collection and information systems.

One option that clearly is not being considered by policymakers is cost-based reimbursement without some type of expenditure control. What seems far more likely is outpatient payment systems with rigorous controls on both volume and per-unit costs and prices. Piecemeal changes moving toward prospective payment systems for outpatient services under Medicare are being introduced at a rapid rate and already can affect the viability of some services.

Although it is impossible to determine the impact of Medicare's recent payment changes, the outcome for tomorrow's payment environment is certain: hospitals must commit strong leadership to keep ambulatory services viable, will require unprecedented managerial innovation, and will require well-designed management information systems to help stimulate such innovations.

The Focus on Outpatient Care

Previously, payment for Medicare outpatient services was done on a cost-reimbursement basis. However, enactment of the Omnibus Budget Reconciliation Act (OBRA) of 1986 has set forth a prospective payment system for all outpatient services by 1991; systems of payment incorporating many features of prospective payment systems already exist for clinical laboratory, ambulatory surgery, and diagnostic radiology services.

Since implementation of the Medicare prospective payment system for inpatient services in 1983, Medicare expenditures for inpatients have slowed considerably while outpatient utilization and expenditures have risen dramatically. In terms of Medicare expenditures for inpatients, costs have risen 35.6 percent from $37.6 billion in 1983 to $51.0 billion in 1988. During the same period, outpatient expenditures have soared 112 percent from $3.3 billion in 1983 to $7.0 billion in 1988. Clearly, with outpatient expenditures now exceeding 10 percent of total Medicare expenditures, policymakers have targeted the ambulatory environment for cost control.

To date, the growth in ambulatory care that has attracted the federal government's attention has prompted a flurry of activity in the development of cost-control strategies. However, attempts to limit cost escalation in the outpatient area have been sporadic and have lacked strong motivation because of the inherent incentives in cost-based reimbursement. Because accounting methods are designed to maximize reimbursement, outpatient "costs" depend on the allocation methods used to distribute costs from nonrevenue- to revenue-producing centers. In addition, cross-subsidization of services occurs within and across departments, with highly profitable services used to subsidize lower charges in other departments. Therefore, cost-based reimbursement has not provided an accurate picture of real resource costs, particularly in outpatient departments. In order to devise cost-control strategies for hospital-based outpatients, hospitals must be able to associate resource use with specific patients and identify their patient mix through a useful case mix classification scheme.

This remaining area of cost-based reimbursement is the one scheduled for change, and once implemented, other payers are likely to follow this payment approach. Currently, the Health Care Financing Administration (HCFA) has funded a number of research projects to develop or evaluate methods of paying for hospital outpatient services using methodologies similar to the inpatient prospective payment system. Although details of the payment system that will emerge from the available research conducted have not been finalized, it is important to understand the findings and implications of the major research that are known.

Outpatient DRG-Like Systems

Although each of the studies funded by HCFA uses a different methodology, they share some common elements. The key similarity is their focus on the patient visit as opposed to an episode of illness. Also, each study combines categories of diseases and, to a certain degree, eliminates the current focus on place of service for reimbursement. Regardless of the specific methodology chosen for an outpatient payment system,

HCFA recognizes the need to reform its current system by creating incentives for efficiency.

Yale University Ambulatory Visit Groups

To date, Medicare system reform of ambulatory care payment has been moving in the direction of establishing a single payment per services or bundle of services, regardless of the setting. Of the methods explored by researchers, ambulatory visit groups (AVGs) first received the greatest interest as the leading prototype for Medicare payment for outpatient services. Developed by the Health Systems Management Group at Yale University, AVGs represent a classification system for ambulatory care patients, using the patient visit as the unit of analysis. This system classifies patients requiring similar patterns of services and consuming comparable quantities of resources into ambulatory visit groups, or AVGs. Ambulatory visit groups have already been used by researchers at Yale and other institutions to measure productivity in ambulatory care and to determine the effect of several variables upon time spent with physicians for certain AVGs.

Ambulatory visit groups are based on the diagnosis related group (DRG) concept also developed at Yale. For AVGs, patients are initially classified into 14 major ambulatory categories (MACs), based on the diagnostic group corresponding to the major organ systems and, in some cases, the specialist involved. The MACs include such categories as "disorders of the nervous system," "diseases of the eye," "accidents, poisons, and violence," and ten others, including a miscellaneous category called "other." Major ambulatory categories were developed using the International Classification of Diseases Adapted for Use in the United States (ICD-8), now updated to the ICD Ninth Revision, Clinical Modification (ICD-9-CM). From these 14 MACs, patients are placed in one of 154 categories, or AVGs.

A decision-tree analysis similar to that used for DRGs determines the ultimate AVG into which a patient falls. Patients are subdivided into AVGs based on resource consumption as determined by physician/provider contact time. Within all the MACs except "other," the first decision point is whether the patient is a "new patient," "revisit/old problem," or "revisit/new problem." Variables used in the subsequent decision process include the major presenting problems, diagnosis, and patient age.

New York State Products of Ambulatory Care

Of the various patient classification schemes funded by HCFA, only one demonstration project—products of ambulatory care (PAC)—has been actually tested in a payment situation. Conducted by the New York State Department of Health since 1987, the PAC payment methodology has been used to reimburse Medicaid patient visits in two geographic areas representing over 20 providers.

The PAC methodology was developed from data on 10,000 outpatients who visited 14 hospitals and 19 diagnostic and treatment centers resulting in over 9,000 observations. From these data, 24 homogeneous payment groups were derived; PACs represent 24 categories of patient visits into which each patient is classified. Patients are assigned to a PAC based on the principal diagnosis of the clinic visit, certain patient characteristics, and the actual services provided to the patient as a result of the visit. There are two broad categories of PACs based on the kinds of services provided: "diagnostic" and "patient management." Diagnostic PACs represent visits in which a diagnostic workup is performed using selected key technologies, such as a CAT scan, whereas management PACs are those for well care or follow-up visits in which no key technologies are provided. Assignment of a patient visit to a PAC is performed by a computer algorithm that classifies a visit based upon age, diagnosis, sex, Current Procedural Terminology—Fourth Edition (CPT-4) procedures, clinic type, provider type, and drug administration.

UCLA Emergency Department Groups

Completed in 1986, emergency department groups (EDGs) were developed at the University of California, Los Angeles, to generate a "relative-value" case mix patient classification scheme for hospital emergency departments. To achieve this case mix system, a large data base consisting of two types of patient-specific information was collected. It contained two kinds of data: (1) patient resource consumption information, from which a standardized measure of resource could be derived; and (2) patient demographic and clinical information, by which patients can be classified. From these data, 216 EDGs from 9 medical diagnostic categories (MDCs) were created. Each MDC is categorized into EDGs according to four variables: disposition of the patient, diagnosis, age of the patient, and procedure performed or injury type. Although constructed on the basis of one dependent variable (measure of total direct cost), each EDG is comprised of two relative values—one for physician care and another for all other hospital direct care services. Thus, EDGs are able to accurately segregate costs of care while also predicting patients' use of ancillary services—unlike AVGs. Despite the fact that EDGs have proven to be a much higher predictor of the overall variance in resource use than AVGs, they have yet to be tested in an automated payment situation, as is being done with PACs in New York State.

Blue Cross of Western Pennsylvania Patient Management Categories

A fourth HCFA-funded study, patient management categories (PMCs), was developed by Blue Cross of Western Pennsylvania, Pittsburgh, to develop a model of integrating hospital inpatient and outpatient reimbursement for cost analysis and for use in hospital reimbursement. Thus, patient categories were derived to identify patient types, or products, treated by hospitals and to identify the relative costs of producing those products.

Although the PMC project encompassed virtually all hospital inpatient types, it has specific utility for ambulatory care patients. Patient management categories can describe the mix of ambulatory patients by general visit types (operative and ancillary) and by more specific categories (procedure-type); identify and describe the volume of inpatient costs that can be effectively managed on an outpatient basis with an examination of the cost implications of reducing the category weight to reflect effective outpatient management; and assess the sensitivity of introducing variation in hospital payments within clinics.

Ambulatory Patient Groups

Although ambulatory visit groups have received the greatest amount of attention, much research is now being devoted to a different type of ambulatory care classification system. This system, ambulatory patient groups (APGs), is based on specific procedures as the primary means of classification, as opposed to DRGs and AVGs, which use diagnosis as the primary point of classification. This fundamental shift has occurred because it has been determined that procedures play a much larger role in predicting resource use than a patient's diagnosis does.

It is anticipated that all outpatient procedures will be divided among approximately 250 APGs. They will be defined based on ICD-9-CM diagnosis codes, CPT procedural codes, age, and sex; will be developed to describe all ambulatory care patients; and will be used across all programmatic settings such as ambulatory surgery, emergency department, clinics, and so forth. Although this new type of classification system will ultimately need approval by Congress, it nevertheless is the favored reimbursement approach for Medicare outpatient services.

Characteristics of a Prospective Payment System

Overall, because a prospective payment system emerging from current methodologies has not yet been adopted, the direction of permanent payment reform appears quantifiable. Similar to the current pricing system for ambulatory surgery, a prospective system for all hospital outpatient services will no doubt have the following characteristics:

1. Payments will be based on fee schedules and will be the same for all providers regardless of facility location.

2. Fees will be all-encompassing, including costs for operating and capital expenditures.
3. Prices will be adjusted only for community wage differences.
4. Payment will increasingly be tied to procedures according to the way physicians bill.
5. Payment will ultimately be made on the basis of an individual episode or "bundle of services."

Impact of Prospective Payment on Ambulatory Care

Regardless of whatever case mix classification is adopted for national implementation in 1991, hospitals will be required to implement operational changes to accommodate the medical records, billing, and other requirements of the evolving payment method. Clearly, information systems capabilities will be an integral component to facilitate such changes.

Case mix systems in ambulatory care are expected to provide decision makers with the product-based information they require for billing, quality assurance, and cost containment in a dynamic environment. In order to control costs for hospital-based outpatients, providers must be able to predict and measure patterns of resource consumption among patients and accurately isolate and define costs within specific services. An essential characteristic of any case mix system is its ability to identify, segregate, and describe a "products" input mix and patient characteristics relevant to that product. Consequently, providers will have to develop clinical, financial, and operational guidelines that capture the requisite payment data and provide a means to measure productivity and ensure efficiency in managing patient care.

Specific Operational Strategies

The following list summarizes the critical success factors that providers must identify and accomplish in order to successfully maneuver their facilities through the prospective payment system schema.

- Capture costs on a per-visit basis.
- Develop ways to associate resource use with specific patients, and identify the mix of patients in terms of the adopted case mix classification scheme.
- Develop product-line costing models that estimate either the total or the per-unit costs of intermediate and end products.
- Prepare to face difficulties in updating, analyzing, and maintaining the requisite data for creating financial and clinical data bases.

- As with inpatient diagnosis related groups, outpatient prospective payment system models will require high-quality data-recording methods. To ensure this, providers must do the following:
  - Overcome the shortage of trained experienced medical record professionals.
  - Develop clearly defined standardized record formats.
  - Work closely with physicians and other patient care providers to ensure that coding and documentation are done with precision and accuracy.
  - Develop training materials for coders.
  - Train billing and medical record personnel in coding and documentation procedures to minimize rejected claims, maximize reimbursement, and improve cash flow.
  - Reevaluate existing practice patterns within the ambulatory care setting because costs will be captured on a per-visit basis.
  - Develop management information systems that provide a "crosswalk" between the inpatient ICD-9-CM codes and the outpatient CPT-4 codes, and develop conversion tables to expedite the interface between these two coding systems.
  - Upgrade present systems and learn about anticipated ambulatory care information systems to increase understanding of the systems' capabilities, and prepare for their future implementation.
  - Relate the costs of providing services with the proposed Medicare reimbursement schedule in order to price services appropriately.
  - Establish reliable data collection systems by focusing on such issues as data verification, data transfer, data entry, data retrieval, and external data validity.
  - Strive to increase volume and spread fixed costs while simultaneously decreasing the costs of supplying services.
  - Investigate ways to restructure ambulatory care services to ensure a predictable revenue stream and minimize economic risk.

Ambulatory Information Systems Requirements

In addition to the operational realities associated with an outpatient prospective payment system, the capture and reporting of key data elements will most likely be necessary to support information systems requirements. Currently, a great deal of attention is being devoted to this endeavor—namely, the development and implementation of a uniform ambulatory medical care data set. Despite the federal government's interest in ambulatory care data, this effort is also being fueled by the ambulatory care data requirements of providers, insurers, and state data commissions who are attempting to develop a comprehensive, integrated outpatient data base for all outpatient programs. Providers are being inundated with requests for data from multiple entities that generally have unique requirements for data reporting. The resultant regulatory reporting burden bears increased costs that are ultimately passed on to the patient. The solution to this growing demand for ambulatory data lies in a nationally recognized and implemented ambulatory data set.

A Uniform Ambulatory Care Data Set

The first recommendation for a uniform ambulatory data set (Uniform Ambulatory Medical Care Data Set, or UAMCDS) was made in 1976 to Congress by a subcommittee of the National Committee on Vital and Health Statistics (NCVHS). Modifications to the original recommendation were proposed in 1981. However, these initial recommendations were shelved for lack of interest. Recent and increasing focus on ambulatory care has prompted the current third effort of the subcommittee to review and update this report. The NCVHS subcommittee appointed to lead this effort held several meetings and submitted a final report in 1989.

The UAMCDS identifies 16 basic patient, provider, and encounter data items that constitute the uniform data set. (These data items are listed in figure 8-1.) This data set contains static and dynamic clinical, financial, and demographic information pertaining to patient, provider, and instance of care. National recognition of a core set of ambulatory data elements allows organizations to expand or enhance their data sets to include additional data elements that may either be unique to their

Figure 8-1. Data Items of the Uniform Ambulatory Care Data Set

Patient Data Items

1. Personal identification
2. Residence
3. Date of birth
4. Sex
5. Race and ethnic background
6. Living arrangement and marital status (optional)

Provider Data Items

7. Provider identification
8. Location or address
9. Profession

Encounter Data Items

10. Date, place, and address of encounter, if different from item 8
11. Patient's reason for encounter (optional)
12. Problem, diagnosis, or assessment
13. Services
14. Disposition
15. Expected source of payment
16. Total charges

environment or necessary for other reporting activities, such as quality assurance.

As stated previously, the data set responds to a number of needs pertinent to the current ambulatory care industry. Areas still requiring discussion and possibly modification in the future include:

- *Encounter definition.* The current definition for *encounter* was developed by both the NCVHS subcommittee and the Interagency Task Force (chaired by HCFA). Both groups have agreed upon the following definition of an ambulatory care encounter: "An ambulatory care encounter is one in which the patient is neither hospitalized nor institutionalized in the facility providing the service at the time of the encounter. An encounter is defined as a face-to-face professional service rendered to a patient by a provider." Discussion over this definition has focused on its emphasis on face-to-face contact with a provider. The subcommittee recommended expanding this definition of encounter to also include a face-to-face professional service rendered to a patient by an individual under the supervision or direction of the provider. This recommended expansion of the definition reflected the subcommittee's sensitivity to inclusion of all instances of ambulatory care in the proposed federal ambulatory care data base.
- *Provider definition.* The 1981 data set defined a *provider* as a health professional who, at some time during the care of the patient, exercises independent judgment. This definition has also been debated, with the main concern being whether the provider is an individual who exercises independent judgment, or an individual who can bill for services rendered. The data set is ambiguous as to whether an encounter has taken place if the prescribing provider is not present. Also of concern is the methodology for accounting for the services of anesthesiologists, pathologists, or radiologists, who provide services in conjunction with other providers.
- *Social security number (SSN).* Should the current data set use the SSN as the common patient identifier? Health Care Financing Administration officials have expressed concern about protecting patient privacy and confidentiality. Because the SSN is currently the common identifier in multiple patient data bases, including patient credit records, its value in the health care arena is great.

It should be noted that the HCFA form 1500 will be the vehicle HCFA will use to support an ambulatory data set. Those involved in the current effort to revise the HCFA data-reporting form 1500 are coordinating with the UAMCDS to achieve consistency on definitions. This interagency cooperation has ensured input from the insurance industry and claims-processing side of HCFA on the appropriate components of a uniform ambulatory data set.

The current lack of comparability among hospitals' outpatient data can be largely attributed to the absence of a uniform definition for *units of service* (encounter/visit/procedure/charge). In addition, coding conventions in ambulatory care vary widely, from diagnostic interpretation on the part of the provider to the actual coding language used (for example, CPT-4, ICD-9-CM). Although more universal use of the CPT-4 coding system is being established via federal reporting mandates, total provider compliance will require significant time and automated system changes, because the ICD-9-CM system has been the coding system most widely used in the ambulatory hospital setting.

Data Collection Issues

Of greatest significance to national imposition of a uniform ambulatory data set is the fact that most hospitals manipulate their ambulatory care data manually. On the basis of this, the question arises as to how ambulatory data can be transmitted, compiled, and reported in a useful and economic manner. The following data-collection and data-extraction issues are associated with the UAMCDS and its potential national implementation:

- *Data verification.* Currently, ambulatory care data are frequently manually coded, with decentralized data collection. Rarely are the clinical and financial data elements integrated. Therefore, providers' ability to verify their ambulatory data is severely limited.
- *Cost-effective data transfer.* Because ambulatory care data are not currently retained in most provider systems, standardized and automated mechanisms must be developed to house, maintain, validate, and report them. Also required is a systematic promulgation of new policies and procedures for both internal management and external agency use.
- *Data entry and retrieval.* Because of the lack of automation in ambulatory care data collection, errors of accuracy and omission occur in data collection and centralized retrieval of data is not possible.
- *Multiplicity of data formats.* Providers are currently responding to several governmental data-reporting requirements that will influence the ways in which inpatient and outpatient data are reported, stored, and collected. At the same time, third-party payers have multiple and differing requirements for patient data, contributing to confusion and frustration in hospital business offices.
- *External data validity.* External data validity is influenced by the following: charge shifting between inpatient and outpatient environments, caseload severity, comparability of data, competitive impact of data, and economic use of the information.

Managing the Current Demand for Data

Although the UAMCDS was initially developed 12 years ago and has since completed its recent modification, sufficient uncertainty exists regarding the final product that many vendors are reluctant to invest significant development efforts in outpatient systems. Rather, many outpatient systems are offshoots or modifications of existing inpatient systems. These systems fall short in their attempts to meet the needs of the ambulatory care arena. Until a standard is implemented, organizations are left to do frequently expensive and labor-intensive improvisation in order to meet the needs of customized requests.

Given the abundance of ambulatory care data and the exploding demand for that data (in as many formats as there are requestors), significant problems have resulted in attempting to form customized responses. Thus, the medical record and information systems departments need to work together to formulate standardized responses where possible. A thorough understanding of the nature and frequency of these requests (both internal and external) will facilitate the development of the most efficient approach for response. For example, comparison of multiple requests may show adequate similarities to justify creation of a standard response that would meet the specific needs of the various requests or the creation of customized reports from a standard response data set. Not only will the standard response data set enable more efficient reporting of data in various customized formats, but the availability of a standard response report may influence the needs of the requestors. It is the responsibility of management to understand the nature of requests for information and to organize those requests based on data requirements that will enable an organization to meet the needs of all requestors despite the lack of a uniform data set and national acceptance of ambulatory care definitions. This ability will also enable an organization to review proposed data sets intelligently and to be positioned favorably when a uniform data set is implemented.

Conclusion

Managerial attention is being increasingly focused on the cost-effective provision of outpatient care. This interest has resulted from a number of factors, the most important being the implementation of DRGs and the rapid initiation of DRG-based payment systems by other payers. In addition, new emerging technologies and the introduction of safer and more effective products have allowed more care to be delivered on an ambulatory basis.

To this end, increasing pressures are being placed on members of the health care delivery system to develop a comprehensive, integrated outpatient data base for all outpatient programs. These pressures are most strongly articulated by the federal government in its progress toward a prospective reimbursement system for ambulatory visits. It is clear that the reimbursement scheme chosen by the federal government and the evolving requirements of entities such as the Joint Commission on Accreditation of Healthcare Organizations will need to be reflected in the outpatient data base that is ultimately adopted by Congress.

Chapter 9

A Review of the Marketplace

Ronald L. Gue and Lawrence D. Visk

The focus of this chapter is various information systems vendors that serve the ambulatory care area. Before turning to the offerings of such vendors, it is helpful to review some aspects of strategic planning such as setting goals, determining needs, and achieving benefits with regard to specific ambulatory service applications.

Information Systems Strategic Planning

Although information systems for ambulatory care are important to many hospitals, our experience indicates that most hospital information systems goals are still focused primarily on inpatient accounting and inpatient care. Competition with other organizations is also a consideration in forming information systems goals and in many cases leads to concentration on computer systems for physician linkages. A large number of hospitals operate in an environment of multiple corporate entities and desire information systems that can support patient care in these complex environments.

As mentioned in chapter 7, achievement of hospital information systems goals is frequently constrained by management's desire to see the investment cost of information systems be offset by quantifiable benefits. Generally, the greatest potential benefits associated with hospital computer expenditures are found in patient accounting and inpatient care. These benefits are usually associated with one of the following:

1. Acute care staff reductions
2. Revenue enhancements
3. Receivable reductions
4. Inventory reductions

The emphasis or importance placed on benefits in information systems planning varies with the style and philosophies of the organization's management. Benefits may only be one factor considered in setting information systems investment priorities. For example, strategic advantage frequently replaces quantifiable benefits as a justification for high priority. In any event, ambulatory service applications are frequently low-benefit areas compared with inpatient care areas.

Information Systems Needs

Hospital information systems needs are most frequently associated with financial and patient care areas such as the following:

- Admitting and registration
- Patient accounting
- General accounting
- Materials management
- Nursing
- Order entry/results reporting
- Ancillaries
- Medical record
- Cost accounting

Within a multientity organization that includes ambulatory services, common registration of, and access to, patient information is a frequently defined need.

In our experience, the most frequently cited ambulatory information system need is hospital linkage with physician offices. Interest in this area is usually for strategic advantage with secondary interest in system functionality, or integration with existing hospital information systems. Other areas receiving attention include physician billing and scheduling, claims processing, home health, outpatient and clinic services, wellness centers, child care, and imaging centers.

Most hospitals see integration of ambulatory information systems with the hospital's information system as important. The most frequent areas of focus are patient registration, billing, and accounts receivable. Integration of physician office systems and the hospital patient data base is extremely important in order not to create unmet expectations and to maintain the competitive advantage that these systems are intended to provide. The value of a computer in the physician's office cannot be fully realized without providing access to information from the inpatient data base such as medication orders and laboratory results. Furthermore, the capabilities of a system without this integration may be quickly met by a competitive system.

Hospital Information Systems

The greatest potential benefit for computer applications in hospitals is in patient care areas, including automation of order entry and patient data retrieval at the nursing station and ancillary department applications. Historically, hospitals have made the largest information system investments in patient accounting. This trend is shifting toward increased investment in patient-related applications and in emerging areas such as patient acuity, nurse scheduling, and dietary. In addition to investing in emerging applications, hospitals are replacing patient accounting and patient care systems where these systems are old and their functionality no longer meets hospital needs.[1,2,3] The demand, internal to the hospital, for investment in inpatient systems is still high. It is in this environment that ambulatory applications must compete for limited information system investment funds.

The Availability of Ambulatory Care Information Systems

Some estimates of the number of companies offering software applications for ambulatory care have been in excess of 1,000. The number of companies is large, and the offerings are diverse and fragmented. A recent listing of ambulatory software vendors by *Computers in Healthcare* contained over 400 companies.[4] This listing was supplemented with information in our files to yield the following summary of the number of companies offering products by major functional area:

Function	Number of Vendors
Outpatient services	150
Group practice appointment scheduling	180
Group practice billing	200
Group practice clinical	140
Home health financial	60
Home health clinical	60
Home health scheduling	50
Durable medical equipment	50
Health maintenance organizations	140
Electronic claims	95
Hospital/physician networking	75

No company listed had offerings in all areas. Most companies had three or fewer offerings. The larger companies specializing in ambulatory information systems are focused on group practice applications.

When attempting to meet the information systems needs of its ambulatory services, hospitals have frequently turned to existing inpatient or outpatient hospital information system software. These attempts have frequently met with problems. Most available systems require a patient to reregister each time the patient enters or uses the ambulatory care system. Many times a bill is generated each time an ambulatory service is provided, leading to patient confusion. Inpatient systems usually cannot post cash collections immediately following a service. Management reporting capabilities of most hospital information systems will not meet the needs of ambulatory services. These and numerous other limitations make hospital information systems software less than satisfactory in meeting the information handling needs of ambulatory services.

The environment in which ambulatory care is provided contains unique information handling challenges not encountered in the typical hospital information systems environment. The patient population served is fragmented, and the services provided are diverse. Patient utilization of ambulatory services is encounter-based, frequently ending with one or two visits. Utilization of ambulatory care resources, including physicians, nurses, equipment, and supplies, has been poor, causing management to look toward information systems for improvements. Increasingly, physician relationships are key to the survival of a hospital and its clinic operations. Many ambulatory services share or create their own ancillary services, or are themselves ancillary services such as retail pharmacies, laboratories, or imaging centers. Many ambulatory services are not covered by insurers, creating complex billing and collection processes.

This chapter is concerned with hospital-focused ambulatory care information systems. In a complete health system network, such as the one shown in figure 9-1, inpatient services could include acute care, long-term care, and hospice services. Ambulatory services could include clinics, physicians in private or group practice, independent ancillary services, such as pharmacy, laboratory, and radiology, managed care such as an HMO, and many other related services such as home health and medical equipment rental. Some hospitals are part of a complete network that contains all of these services and others. Many hospitals relate to only a portion of these ambulatory services. In any case, the most commonly cited needs in such an environment are for common patient registration capabilities, for access to the patient record for all elements of the health system network, and for the need to link physicians to a common patient data base. Although a number of vendors have such systems in development, a system that provides these capabilities to a complete health system network does not exist.

Among the elements of a complete health systems network as shown in figure 9-1, information systems to support acute patient care and clinic operations are the highest-priority areas in the health system. These

Figure 9-1. A Complete Health Care System Network

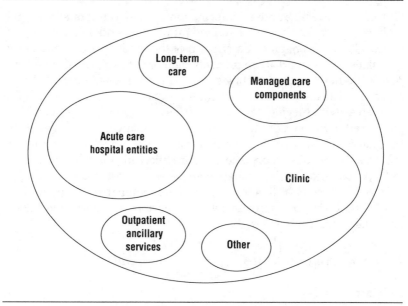

two areas have received the greatest portion of vendor research and development expenditures and represent the largest portion of health care information systems expenditure. For the most part, a different set of vendors have pursued the acute care market than have focused on the clinic market. This means that current ambulatory information systems expenditures are largely concentrated on clinic and group practice operations. In addition, there is limited integration between acute care systems and clinic information systems or among ambulatory information systems in general.

Although integrated systems for linking acute care systems, clinic operations, and other ambulatory services are not available, hospitals continue to move toward meeting their ambulatory information systems needs. Their strategies in meeting these needs fall into one of the following categories:

1. Developing their own information systems for ambulatory services
2. Adding ambulatory care modules to their current inpatient systems
3. Purchasing standalone systems to meet specific ambulatory information system needs

The most frequent investment in standalone systems is in linking the physician's office to the patient data base.

Major Players in the Marketplace

Out of the several hundred information system vendors serving the ambulatory services market, a limited number of vendors were selected to include in this chapter's description of the marketplace. Many of the companies in the market are privately held or subsidiaries of large companies. In these cases, operating statistics on revenue, number of clients, and other data are difficult to obtain. Information was solicited from the companies with varying degrees of success. Telephone interviews were conducted with most of these companies. In many cases, clients of the companies were contacted to verify information and to enlarge our perspective. Using this information, information in our files, and other industry sources, market leaders were selected. In the discussion that follows, the results of this investigation are summarized. Appendix A provides a listing of approximately 140 vendors that appear to have a nationally focused business base.

Principal Ambulatory Care Software Vendors

AISCorp
In 1987, AIS recorded $8 million in revenues from approximately 200 clients. In the past, the company's products focused on the small to medium-sized group practice markets operating on DEC PDP and Vax hardware. Some clients are served on a shared basis. In 1988, the company entered into a marketing arrangement with IBM to modify its product for the AS/400. As a result, it stopped selling its product for DEC installations. The AS/400 version of the product should allow the company faster growth in the large group practice and educational facility practice markets.

Annson Systems Division, Baxter Corporation
Baxter's Annson Systems Division is a separate division independent of the Baxter Information Systems Division, a leading industry provider of hospital information systems. Annson's product line is concentrated on solo practice and small to medium-sized group practices. It also markets a product that allows the linking of its physicians' product with a hospital information system. The Annson Doctors Office Management System (DOMS) is designed for use on IBM personal computers by small group practices and solo practice physicians. This product is available under an IBM label and may even be purchased in retail computer stores. There are approximately 7,000 users of DOMS, 3,000 of which are Annson clients. The remainder purchased the software through IBM or third parties. Annson software operates on IBM personal computers and DEC MicroVax computers.

Annson also markets their Exchange product, which allows physician-to-physician and physician-to-hospital communication. This is an example of the physician link product mentioned earlier in the chapter. Annson is also working on a physician-to-HMO and an HMO-to-hospital link.

APS Systems, Inc.

APS is a publicly owned company that had approximately $12 million in revenue in 1987. The company has three divisions. The Malpractice Division is concerned with insurance administration. The Financial Services Division designs and supports 401K plans, pension programs, and related services. The APS Systems Division provides data-processing services, primarily to group practices. APS Systems accounted for approximately 30 percent of total revenues for APS in 1987.

In February 1988, APS sold its Data Bill Division to CyCare, reducing its annual revenues from $30 million to the present level of $12 million. Data Bill had 1,500 clients concentrated in the small and group practice market. The resulting focus of the APS Systems Division is on large group practices and on medical teaching facility groups. They will provide their services as in-house turnkey systems, shared services, or as a total facility management, assuming all responsibility for system maintenance and operation. APS software runs on the HP 3000 series.

CyCare Systems, Inc.

CyCare specializes in software for physicians' office operations and is the leader in this market, with approximately 5,500 clients. Its client base ranges from solo practice physicians to large group practices with a hundred or more physicians. In 1987, their total revenues were approximately $68 million. CyCare has experienced significant internal growth, but most recently has made a number of acquisitions that have also contributed to growth. For example, in 1986 the company acquired Data Bill Division of the APS Group, Inc., which brought 1,500 new small group practice clients to the business. In 1988, the company entered the hospital information systems market by acquiring the financial and patient care systems developed by Carraway Methodist Hospital in Birmingham, Alabama.

CyCare uses a number of delivery modes to provide software to its customer. These include batch, remote batch, shared processing, distributed processing, and in-house turnkey systems. During the past two years, CyCare has reorganized its customer support activity, resulting in unrest among its customers. During the same period, it converted its Honeywell-based large group practice software product to IBM. This has also created some unrest among its large group practice clients. Overall, the company is financially strong and growing. Resolution of some of its growing pains is required for continued growth and maintenance of its market share.

Healthserv, Inc.

Healthserv's 1987 revenues were $20 million from over 300 clients in small and medium-sized group practices. The company's focus is on accounts receivable and collection for hospital-based specialty groups. Delivery modes include facilities management and in-house turnkey systems, with facilities management making up 70 percent of its clients. The company's growth strategy is concentrated on acquisition of other companies whose clients it would convert to its own software. Healthserv software runs on NCR, Prime, and Micro Data hardware.

IDX Corporation
IDX is a privately held corporation that had approximately $45 million in revenues in 1987. Sixty-five percent of its revenues come from the ambulatory care market. It has a total of approximately 600 clients, about 150 of which are in ambulatory information systems. IDX's target markets are large freestanding clinics and group practices, university-based practices, managed care plans, and hospital-based outpatient facilities. Its group practice products are focused on large and small group practices. These products use Digital Equipment Corporation (DEC) hardware.

Medic Computer Systems
Medic Computer Systems, a subsidiary of Emhart Corporation, has approximately 2,000 clients, which generated approximately $40 million in revenue in 1987. The company offers its products to medical clinics, group practices, and solo practitioners. Its focus is on practices with 1 to 50 practitioners. Medic software runs on Texas Instruments 1000 series and IBM personal computers.

National Medical Computer Services, Inc.
National Medical Computer Services (NMCS), a division of Reynolds & Reynolds, had over 1,000 client installations in 1987, producing approximately $25 million in revenue. The company's focus is on hospital-based specialty group practices with their Physicians Accounts Receivable (PAR) product. National Medical Computer Services also has a practice management module, which it sells to group practices with a recurring patient population. Specialized system modules are offered to pathologists, radiologists, anesthesiologists, cardiologists, and virologists. Their focus is on group practices with 5 to 10 members. However, a current effort to convert current software to the IBM AS/400 will allow them to sell to large group practices.

The company also has a radiology management system, which it intends to sell to diagnostic imaging centers rather than hospitals. Delivery modes for NMCS software include in-house turnkey, facilities management, and shared service, with in-house turnkey systems making up approximately 90 percent of the company's revenue.

Science Dynamics
Science Dynamics is a privately held company that had approximately $12 million in revenue in 1987. The company was acquired by McDonnell

Douglas Automation in 1984 and sold back to its employees in early 1988. The company currently has approximately 350 clients. Its two principal products are focused on small and medium-sized group practices. Their software currently runs on IBM personal computers, DEC Vax, and MicroVax. The company has versions under development for the IBM AS/400 and the Hewlett-Packard (HP) 3000. The company previously offered its software as a shared service. However, current efforts are to convert these shared clients to in-house operation.

Shared Medical Systems (SMS)

Shared Medical Systems is the hospital information system market leader, with over 800 hospital clients. Shared Medical Systems' Physician Services Division offers two products to the group practice market. The Signature product is directed toward large group practices and medical teaching facilities. Its Physicians Office System is directed toward small group practices and solo practice physicians. Shared Medical Systems also continues to support its Physicians Billing System, which was developed in the 1970s. The Signature product is relatively new, having been first installed in a medical teaching facility in 1985.

Shared Medical Systems' hardware strategy in this market is focused on IBM with Signature using mainframes and the Physicians Office System using microcomputers. Signature is offered using SMS's remote computing option (RCO), where computer equipment is located at an SMS client site linked by telephone lines or satellite communications to the group practice client. Shared Medical Systems claims to be headed toward integration of the Signature product with its mainframe-based hospital information systems. They have made some progress in this area with common patient registration capability operating in several client sites. The principal focus of future SMS product development will continue to be in hospital information systems. Product development investment in ambulatory systems will be secondary to hospital information systems and could be expected to complement and support its hospital information system product strategy.

Principal Hospital Information Systems Vendors

The leaders of the hospital information systems market have varying strategies related to ambulatory information systems. None of the market leaders have made a strong commitment to this market, including group practice physicians.

Baxter has entered the ambulatory care market through its Annson Systems Division. A substantial portion of its current product development effort is committed to its Exchange product, which links the physician's office to the hospital data base. Although they have identified a fully integrated hospital-ambulatory services product as a future objective, their current software offerings are not there yet.

HBO & Company has no announced plans to actively enter the clinic or group practice market. In 1988, they sold their interest in Computer Resources, Inc., a company selling software for home health services. HBO has incorporated several design considerations for hospital out-patients in its new Star series of products. In addition, they offer resource scheduling and physician link capabilities to their hospital clients.

McDonnell Douglas developed an ambulatory care practice system that never succeeded as a standalone product. Subsequently, it added the functionality of this software to its HFC system for hospitals. This is now an option in its HFC financial system. The functionality of its hospital systems has also been enhanced to meet the increased demands of outpatient processing.

Shared Medical Systems has recently improved the functionality of its hospital software to support outpatient processing. It entered the group practice market through its Signature and Physicians' Office System. It claims to have an ambulatory clinical system under development, using its inpatient care system as a base. Although SMS has made some progress in integrating its hospital and ambulatory products—for example, patient registration—it needs to develop further synergies between its Hospital and Physician Services divisions.

Ambulatory Care Vendors Entering the Hospital Information Systems Market

Two ambulatory system vendors, CyCare and IDX, have seriously entered the hospital information systems market.

CyCare entered the hospital information systems market by acquiring a system developed by Carraway Methodist Hospital in Birmingham, Alabama. The acquired software included complete financial systems and order entry/results reporting. CyCare's initial attempts to integrate the Carraway software with their large group practice system has suffered delays. Turnover in the newly formed Hospital Division has created further difficulties. At this time the combined integrated system is still under development and not fully operational.

IDX has used acquired and internally developed systems to enter the medium-sized hospital market. It currently claims 18 hospital information system clients. Its product offerings include financial systems, order entry/results reporting, radiology, laboratory, and a pharmacy system under development. The company claims that 10 of its hospital clients have integrated its hospital and group practice systems through use of a common patient data base.

Summary of Software Vendors

Several hundred vendors offer one or more software products or services to the ambulatory services market. This market is highly fragmented. Many vendors offer only one product and restrict their business activity to only one region of the country. Very few vendors offer most products to the market. Many vendors have grown through acquisition of smaller companies. In some cases, this has resulted in disjointed product offerings and customer support.

Very few vendors have revenues over $10 million, and few have a truly national focus. The largest vendors receive most of their revenues from sales related to physician group practice. Although many companies offer software in other ambulatory services such as home health and durable medical equipment, this represents a minor portion of the expenditures in the market. The evolution of ambulatory software is following a pattern similar to the evolution of hospital software. Initial attention has been on financial systems with concentration on clinical systems coming later. Physician link capability is used by many hospitals as a first step toward a computerized health care system network. Integration of available and future products is needed, but this is years away.

Principal Hardware Vendors

For the most part the hardware vendors supplying the hospital information systems market have not aggressively pursued the ambulatory care market. All have developed relationships with value added retailers (VARs) or companies who develop, sell, and install software to operate on a particular vendor's hardware. The following descriptions briefly summarize hardware vendor activities:

Data General Corporation: Data General Corporation provides no proprietary software for ambulatory systems. The following are some of the VAR relationships that it has with ambulatory software vendors:

- Epic Systems
- Ciphor Corporation
- Elcomp
- Paul Marc Systems

Digital Equipment Corporation: Digital Equipment Corporation has no proprietary software for ambulatory care. It has been active in establishing third-party marketing relationships. Selected vendors with which it has such relationships include the following:

- Calyx Corporation
- Execu-Flow Systems, Inc.
- Global Health Systems, Inc.
- IDX Corporation
- Shared Medical Systems

Hewlett-Packard: Hewlett-Packard has no software for ambulatory care systems and sells its hardware through VARs. Principal VAR relationships include the following:

- PSI-MED
- MOS
- Global Health Systems, Inc.
- Westland Software
- APS Group, Inc.
- Science Dynamics

IBM: IBM has no proprietary software that it sells in the ambulatory systems market. It does have a variety of marketing relationships with third parties, including over 50 VARs. AS/400 VARs include the following:

- National Medical Computer Services
- AISCorp
- Information Systems of North Carolina
- Millard Wayne

Other third-party vendors use IBM personal computers.

NCR: NCR provides no proprietary software to the ambulatory systems market. It has preferred marketing relationships with selected vendors including:

- Disc Based Computer Systems
- Wallaby Systems

Unisys: Unisys is the only major hardware vendor to offer proprietary software to the ambulatory systems market. It markets the Total Practice Management Solution to the group practice market. It has approximately 30 clients for this product, most of which are small group practices. It also has plans to develop a hospital–physician link. Unisys also has third-party relationships with several software vendors including:

- Calyx Corporation
- Experior Corporation
- Medical Computer Management, Inc.
- Keystone Technology, Inc.

Summary of Vendors

Unisys is the only major hardware vendor to develop and sell proprietary software in the ambulatory information systems market. All major vendors have established third-party marketing relationships in the market. These marketing relationships extend beyond group practice applications to other ambulatory care markets including home health, mental health, and managed care. IBM's AS/400 series has provided the opportunity and incentive for many software vendors to extend their group practice offerings to larger groups.

Conclusion

Most ambulatory applications are not a high priority in hospital information system strategic plans. In those hospitals where ambulatory applications are important, integration of ambulatory systems with the patient data base is a critical success factor. Common patient registration and physician links seem to be the highest-priority ambulatory applications. Both these applications should be integrated with the patient data base.

Many ambulatory applications are personal-computer applications requiring limited capital investment for product development. This has provided the opportunity for many new companies to enter the market. Very few of these vendors have a national client base or revenues in excess of $10 million. The largest vendors serve the group practice market, to which they offer very comprehensive products.

The major hospital information systems suppliers have made a limited commitment to the market and seem to be waiting for further development. Two group practice vendors have made a major commitment to the hospital information systems market. They are attempting to use their group practice business as a foundation for entry.

The ambulatory information systems market is highly fragmented and is concentrated on the group practice segment of the market. However, in the case of hospital-based ambulatory services, required expenditures must compete with inpatient financial and patient care applications for limited capital resources. In the near term, hospital information systems capital expenditures will not tend to be shifted in a significant way to ambulatory services.

References

1. Packer, C. L. Info systems critical to 1989 planning, success. *Hospitals* 63(2): 76, Jan. 20, 1989.

2. Dorenfest, S. I. Hospitals are ripe for replacing many patient accounting systems. *Modern Healthcare* 18(36), Sept. 2, 1988.

3. *Profile Fact Book.* New York City: McGraw-Hill, 1988.

4. *Computers in Healthcare, 1988 Market Directory.* Cardiff Publishing Co.

Part Two

Applications for Patient Care

Chapter 10

Ambulatory Surgery

Theodore A. Matson

Each ambulatory care program or service has its own critical information needs, and this is particularly true for ambulatory surgery. In addition to providing for the data processing and information handling capabilities to support patient registration, order entry, test processing, and results storage, secondary support capabilities are imperative as well. These include maintaining patient history information, accurately assigning coding and billing information, and performing departmental statistical reporting.

Because of the unique needs of ambulatory surgery patients, it is important to review the management process of these cases in order to demonstrate specific information systems requirements that may be necessary. Issues related to hospital-based ambulatory surgery programs will be illustrated because they represent approximately 85 percent of the outpatient surgical marketplace. After the management process has been described, specific requirements for patient registration, resource/service scheduling, and statistical reporting will be covered.

Ambulatory Surgery Management Process

The popularity of ambulatory surgery, fueled by improvements in surgical techniques, technological developments, and cost concerns, is most evident in the overwhelming interest expressed by patients and providers. Despite the tremendous growth in procedures performed and the multitude of physical settings that are now available, patients undergoing ambulatory surgery are very satisfied with their experiences. In addition, satisfaction from physicians is also quite high.

These attitudes reflect the very reasons why ambulatory surgery is so pervasive today. Because most procedural cases are elective, efficiency in treating cases is achieved. Patients are selected carefully, and the actual surgical management of patients is routine. Because accurate time estimates for treating cases can be made, operating rooms and physicians' surgical time can be scheduled in specific time periods to minimize downtime between cases. In addition, cancellations and overlap of the time blocks for various cases are almost nonexistent.

Therefore, much of the effort required for effective management of the surgical process is done prior to the actual day of surgery. Patients must be briefed on the surgery in an interview and educational session, where they receive instructions about the prepreparation and the actual procedure(s). On average, all items related to the patient's surgery must be available in the medical chart at the facility approximately 48 hours before surgery. This information includes a preoperative history and physical, preanesthesia evaluation, and preanesthesia testing (for example, laboratory tests, X rays, EKGs, and so forth).

Once patients have complied with all preoperative requests, they must register with the facility to ensure that all pertinent demographic, billing, and other data requirements are satisfied. In many instances, patients are preregistered well in advance of the surgery date, and this information is again confirmed 90 minutes before the operating time. After the surgical procedure(s) is completed, a recovery period of two to three hours begins and the patient is subsequently discharged or (in rare instances) admitted.

In the past few years, many facilities have been experiencing an increase in the mix of patients who require extended hours for recovery (for example, six to eight hours). This results primarily from newer procedures that previously were done on an inpatient basis and from the increasing proportion of patients with chronic illnesses. It is predicted that extended-recovery patients will soon represent a large number of surgical patients as technological advances allow more of these procedures to be performed. This will pose a great challenge for hospitals because significant operational, financial, and human resources will be required. Information systems will play a substantial role in supporting these developments.

Information Systems Requirements

As indicated previously, ambulatory surgery programs have a distinct advantage over other ambulatory services because their patients are scheduled in advance, generally have all tests performed prior to the day of surgery, and rarely cancel. This pragmatic approach, unfortunately, has not led to widespread industry development of information systems for ambulatory surgery. Some facilities do not perceive that a need exists for such immediate on-line order entry, results reporting, and other functions. Also, because the majority of programs are integrated within the hospital's main operating room suites, scheduling of patients and rooms may be done independent of the ambulatory surgery program and compiled manually. Recent developments in ambulatory surgery have included systems being built for certain automated functions; however, they are often configured to the unique needs and desires of each facility.

In the future, full-scale automation will be imperative because ambulatory growth will necessitate state-of-the-art systems that increase the operational and managerial processing of all outpatient and inpatient surgical cases. To this end, comprehensive systems for ambulatory surgery that incorporate specific functional requirements may include but not be limited to the following: preregistration and outpatient registration, including patient history profiles; resource/service scheduling; and statistical reporting.

Preregistration/Testing

The purpose of the preregistration process is to decrease the length of time required to register patients. It serves as a preliminary indicator of expected utilization of a program or service. Originally developed exclusively for inpatient admissions, it has since been expanded to meet the growing numbers and complexities associated with outpatients.

When a patient is scheduled for an ambulatory surgical procedure, he or she is sent a computer-generated preregistration form that contains vital patient demographic and billing information. Data elements include the following items for each patient:

- Name
- Age
- Address
- Telephone number
- Date of birth
- Assigned history number
- Previous history number, if applicable
- Preadmission number
- Insurance carrier information
- Physician(s)
- Date and time of scheduled surgery
- Billing codes
- Preregistration testing date, time, and orders

This process generally occurs when a procedure is scheduled one week or more in advance; shorter scheduling dates will require this information to be obtained by telephone (or done at the time of outpatient registration/testing).

The ultimate benefit, therefore, is derived when all data are stored and then updated at the time of formal outpatient registration. Prior to this event, any discrepancies noted can be corrected, thus ensuring the efficiency of the surgery management process.

Outpatient Registration

The purpose of the outpatient registration process is to ascertain pertinent information and assign a patient number to individuals who receive services on an outpatient basis. As indicated previously, if patients have provided demographic information via the preregistration process, it is merely verified and updated as appropriate.

When formal outpatient registration does occur, past information in the history profile can be accessed by various departments via the communications, order entry, and results-reporting function. Although testing information is normally given to the attending physician no later than 48 hours prior to the procedure, some routine testing is performed and reviewed the morning of surgery; previous testing is verified at this time as well.

The outpatient registration function is extremely important, obviously, because it creates the central component of the surgical process. Because this vital information is stored, statistical reporting of various data elements allows for forecasting and modeling of surgical cases. Any changes in utilization, physician practice patterns, and reimbursement can be analyzed to enhance managerial/clinical decision making.

Resource/Service Scheduling

In addition to outpatient registration, ambulatory surgery patients will require departmental scheduling for various tests and operating room services. To perform these functions, a resource/service scheduling function is required. Using the scheduled procedure date and time, its purpose is to notify the appropriate departments that certain activities need to be performed. For instance, this function should facilitate scheduling of specific operating rooms by attending physician and blocks of time routinely allocated to physicians according to number of patients, procedure(s) planned, estimated time by procedure, anesthesia required, and nursing personnel required. Because hospital-based ambulatory surgery is generally integrated within the existing operating room suites, the system should have the capability to incorporate the scheduling of outpatient procedures that are always performed in inpatient surgery suites and inpatient procedures always performed in ambulatory surgery rooms. A system of this nature should also recommend a procedure room based on certain parameters such as physician room preference and planned procedure(s), patient diagnosis, and availability of facility rooms and specialized equipment.

Statistical Reporting

Currently, a large portion of ambulatory care data is manually reported in most institutions. Unfortunately, ambulatory care suffers in this regard; profound changes occurring in the industry will require sophisticated data collection and reporting to effectively manage these departments. Ambulatory surgery in particular requires significant amounts of data to accurately predict utilization and reimbursement changes that are forthcoming with the advent of a fully prospective payment system mandated to occur in 1991 by the Health Care Financing Administration.

A statistical reporting system ultimately required for ambulatory surgery should provide for individual and cumulative collection and reporting of the various volumes of work provided. Specifically, a system should report statistics according to ambulatory surgery procedures by ICD-9-CM and CPT-4 codes; associated anesthesiology procedures by class type; ancillary tests for groups of procedures to identify case mix profiles; units of production/service; identifiable relative value units such as physician and facility resource consumption; and operating room utilization according to procedures performed, hours utilized per room, hours utilized by room and physician, hours by attending medical specialty, total number of cases by procedure, canceled cases, and cases requiring subsequent inpatient admission. In addition, operational parameters such as work load and other productivity measures are important to monitor, control, and forecast departmental output.

Conclusion

Ambulatory surgery information systems are receiving more emphasis than other systems for ambulatory care, despite the absence of these developments in the marketplace, literature, and trade journals. This emphasis, however, relates to efforts of various components of the ambulatory surgery process such as operating room scheduling. Medical records and billing functions, issues beyond the scope of this discussion, often continue to be contained in existing functional areas of each institution's overall information systems. As the complexities increase for ambulatory surgery applications, it is probable that dedicated information systems capabilities will be necessary. Systems of this nature will need to incorporate all phases of the surgery management process from preregistration and testing to medical records documentation and patient billing. Until these decentralized programs are developed, a true "service-line" approach directed at the management and operation of ambulatory surgery programs cannot be fully realized.

Chapter 11

Emergency Department

Theodore A. Matson

Until recently, information systems for the emergency department consisted merely of outpatient registration and financial management components. Generally, these applications were part of the traditional hospital information system or developed as part of an in-house system.

In recent years, system functionality has been expanded to include many items:

- Complex registration capabilities
- Patient flow monitoring
- Clinical uses including reference information retrieval, automated diagnoses based upon symptoms, and other clinical parameters
- Drug dosage calculations
- Patient history profiles
- Medical records management, including system-driven and voice-activated report dictation
- Trauma registries
- Point-of-service billing
- External facility linkages
- Automated patient discharge instructions

Although available in various forms and configurations, highly complex systems incorporating all of these features are not yet readily available. Applications are very much in their infancy and will continue to undergo numerous revisions, testing, and demonstrations before they are considered as serious acquisitions by hospitals.

This situation is unfortunate, because the emergency department is perhaps the one hospital outpatient department experiencing the greatest and most immediate need for comprehensive information systems processing. Overall, it usually represents the single largest outpatient department in terms of patient encounters on any given day; nearly 100 percent of patients are not scheduled and thus truly classified as "walk-ins." The emergency department accounts for a substantial portion of other ancillary department utilization (for example, radiology, laboratory, and so forth), and it is increasingly complex to manage in terms of expanding patient loads, acuity levels, and the efficient processing of all patient care data. In short, it is becoming nearly impossible to satisfy the operational demands of today's emergency department without dedicated information systems tailored to the unique needs of each emergency department patient. As hospitals begin their planning efforts for improved automation in the emergency department setting, many will find that they will either forgo purchasing information products and services until such systems are ready for marketplace distribution or will attempt shorter-term solutions via in-house developments or modifications to existing system capabilities. Regardless, the outcome of these events will no doubt consist of a highly complex on-line, real-time information processing system. Although each institution will have individual information needs, the following overview highlights system components and features that most hospitals will desire as standard functional requirements for an emergency department information system.

Outpatient Registration

The extremely high volume of unscheduled emergency department patients requires the collection of numerous data elements within a short time period. Historically, most hospitals have required a minimal amount of data at the time of patient registration. Name, age, address, sex, physician information, and insurance/payer information were the only core requirements. This philosophy has now changed dramatically with the number of managed care plans and restrictive patterns of insurers that require complex recordkeeping for reimbursement purposes; administrative needs for statistical reporting; state-mandated requirements for specialized categorical programs, such as burn and trauma care; quality assurance and peer review activities; and the need to generate complex billing statements for payment at time of services rendered. Clearly, some information systems were not designed for these needs and often cannot be modified to the extent now required.

To comply with today's complex data needs, additional items must be captured at the time of registration. They include the type of patient (return patient, series, referred from another outpatient department, and so forth); mode of arrival, including prehospital care provider by name and address; detailed data concerning financial status; data for multiple insurance companies and policy numbers; managed care plan(s) with necessary detail such as visit eligibility; and expanded physician information such as referring, transferring, and consulting physician(s).

These data elements, however, must be available on-line, real-time, if they are to be fully maximized. Once captured, they form the integral portion of the patient record; tests are requested and bills generated quickly as elements are transferred from one application to another. In addition, with sophistication, a system can track the patient's course of treatment from initial registration, triage, ancillary testing, and pending hospital admission to final disposition, with subsequent time intervals posted for each activity. This creates unique profiles for each patient and yields data on patient type, waiting times for individual ancillary procedures and reporting of results, physician consults, and admission to each inpatient type unit. Combined with productivity and staffing measures, this information can greatly enhance operational decision making.

Patient Care Management

A real-time, on-line information system has many distinct advantages for patient care compared with existing information systems. At registration or triage, a unique patient numbering system allows for immediate cathode ray tube (CRT) inquiry to patient history profiles. Previous visits to the department, test results, diagnosis, and disposition instructions are evaluated quickly to expedite the treatment regimen of each patient.

Specific functions of this system allow for the ability to properly identify past patients according to multiple search criteria such as patient name, maiden name, date of birth, and social security number. Also, access is immediate to previous inpatient and outpatient medical encounters by diagnosis, physician, and service; problem lists; and ancillary tests performed as both an inpatient and outpatient. Other demographic and financial data elements are easily identified according to insurance carrier by name, codes, and policy numbers as well.

In terms of clinical needs, sophisticated information systems can incorporate many interesting capabilities. Excluding a totally automated medical record (which is beyond the scope of this discussion), common uses include clinical reference information retrieval and programs that allow interpretation of specific patient information. For instance, reference retrieval is accessed to yield toxicology ingestions and treatments (poison control information). Other examples include programs that perform drug dosage calculations, drug-to-drug interactions, and artificial intelligence systems (which provide clinical diagnosis interpretations or possibilities from various patient signs and symptoms).

Another patient care management function now desired by institutions is the immediate on-line terminal inquiry to the inpatient admitting system. The emergency department, as the largest admitting source for hospitals, is now considered the short-stay or observation unit for patients awaiting hospital admission when inpatient beds are not readily available. Thus, with increasing patient volumes, the emergency department must expedite the transfer and admission of patients via the inpatient admitting system. Historically, patient admissions were handled by the admitting department, but the complexities of today's emergency department admissions often require this decentralized function to be placed in the emergency department as well.

To properly facilitate such transfers from the emergency department, real-time, on-line terminal inquiry must be available. At the time of admission, a system should automatically provide patient information previously stored in the outpatient registration file; generate the patient's record; and communicate all pertinent information to the hospital's departments and services. Ideally, this system should also provide an audit trail of the patient's location from the emergency department admission through the entire hospital stay. Because of the emergency department's need to ensure continuity of patient transfers, unique system capabilities are also necessary. For instance, a system should have the ability for the receiving nursing unit to confirm on-line that a patient has arrived, find out the patient's status and type of arrival, and confirm any outstanding items ordered in the emergency department (such as tests) that have not yet been received.

A final function required in the emergency department for improved patient care management is in the area of medical records management. A number of patients revisit the emergency department, some within several days after a previous visit and some after more than one year. Regardless, they may have complex and chronic medical conditions that require abstracting of the actual medical record for review and consultation. With the ability to review on-line, patient-specific information from the medical record, the management process can be greatly enhanced. Although it may be impossible to have access to a complete medical record, certain data from medical charts can be captured and stored on-line for one year and off-line thereafter via a computer-readable medium. A list of abstract data commonly referenced or desired is shown in figure 11-1.

Point-of-Service Billing

The financial management and reimbursement maximization in the emergency department setting has recently incorporated a new philosophy of seeking payment at time of services rendered. Although many emergency departments have often asked or encouraged patients for payment, immediate payment is readily becoming a requirement. Often, emergency department visits can generate $200 to $300 in average

Figure 11-1. Medical Record Abstract Data Commonly Referenced

Patient Identification
Hospital identification number
Medical record number
Patient name, age, sex, address, birthdate

Outpatient Visit History
Visit date, hour, and department(s)
Disposition and hour
Attending physician(s)
Consulting physician(s)
Operating physician(s)
Principal diagnoses
Secondary diagnoses
Principal procedures
Ancillary tests and results
Admission date, hour, unit (if applicable)

Inpatient Visit History
Admission date and hour
Attending physician(s)
Consulting physician(s)
Operating physician(s)
Principal diagnoses
Secondary diagnoses
Principal procedure(s)
Ancillary tests and results
Medical service code
Special service unit type
Severity index (classification)

Source: Division of Ambulatory Care and Health Promotion, American Hospital Association, 1989.

patient charges, which increasingly are subject to scrutiny by payers as to what constitutes an appropriate and reimbursable visit. In addition, expanding volumes of uninsured patients, which cause per-unit charges to increase for insured patients, and the lack of payment from managed care plans for treatment rendered but not authorized are causing the collection of patient receivables to reach unacceptable levels.

Because the emergency department may be the only source of contact for patients, it is here that the accurate capture and verification of insurance information or receipt of payment must be performed. In terms of data capture, along with previous demographic elements, a system must be capable of assigning CPT-4 coding to all procedures performed. With this information and ICD-9-CM diagnosis coding, a complete facility bill can be printed and verified immediately after patient discharge. Generally, unless specific payer or insurer information and eligibility can be verified, patients are requested to pay via check or credit card. This is particularly important for patients covered under managed care plans—many simply will not reimburse for patient care in the emergency department, whether medically or nonmedically justified. Overall, these scenarios are vastly different from previous documentation and collection methods, yet they represent the stark reality of ensuring payment for reimbursement for emergency department services. Some institutions will find they have no other alternative than to pursue this approach.

Statistical Reporting

The emergency department is highly dependent on timely, accurate data for decision-making purposes. Aside from patient care activities, a large portion of data can be collected and reported to observe changes in patient mix, physician referrals, and transferring institutions, and it can be utilized for planning new programs and service offerings. Without this information, management decisions can be highly inaccurate.

For each emergency department patient, a large number of data elements must be stored and available via a flexible report-writing capability that is user-friendly. For certain categories of patients (general medical, cardiac, poisoning, motor-vehicle trauma, and so forth), profiles of all resources expended to patients should be available. Thus, all cardiac patients treated in the emergency department should be profiled according to method of arrival, time of day, day of week, time at triage, time in treatment room, initial physical and history, test(s) ordered, treatment regimen, time to cardiology consult, time to intensive care unit admission, and related patient demographics. This information allows for observing patients and their care over time and is the basis for expanding the types of services offered and those available.

With sophisticated patient profiles, an institution can accurately predict the overall hospital's dependence on the activities of the emergency department—for example, its laboratory and radiology testing capabilities and performance. This is particularly valuable when departmental volumes increase substantially, when changes in patient mix occur, and when the need to improve profit margins through productivity monitoring is required.

External Hospital Links

In the future, comprehensive information links will be a necessity between acute care hospitals and physician offices, affiliated hospital networks, and rural hospital emergency departments. As technological capabilities and patient care needs change, these links will serve as the central component of health care delivery among settings. Several scenarios highlight the complexities of such linkages. For instance, a patient may first visit a private physician's office for chest pain. Upon further analysis, it is deemed necessary that the patient be transferred to an emergency department for a more thorough diagnostic workup. Having previously stored vital information at registration, the emergency department accesses the patient history profile maintained on-line and requests immediate retrieval of the patient's medical record. After initial review and consultation between transferring and receiving physician, all conducted prior to and during transit of the patient, a cardiologist is immediately consulted and requests certain tests and procedures upon patient arrival.

In some instances, patients may be treated in the emergency department or go directly to the cardiovascular department or catheterization laboratory, or perhaps immediately to an operating room suite.

A similar situation can and probably will exist for emergency departments that have 24-hour links to hospitals in their tertiary services network or affiliations in staffing small or rural hospitals. In any event, patient care scenarios will be similar; information-handling capabilities will greatly facilitate the delivery of services for patients between two facilities. Much of these developments will be in tandem with sophisticated telemetry, digital transmission, and other voice communication capabilities; yet dedicated information systems will comprise the focal point of such efforts.

Conclusion

Because emergency departments need immediate access to many kinds of patient data, a comprehensive, on-line, real-time information system has many advantages over other kinds of information systems. An emergency department information system must be able to provide data for outpatient registration, patient care management, point-of-service billing, and statistical reporting and may also need to be linked to other external hospital systems.

Chapter 12

Radiology Department

Theodore A. Matson

Radiology services provided by hospitals represent one of the fastest-growing areas of outpatient care. Competition and technological advances have created new and improved imaging modalities that were nonexistent 10 years ago. This growth has also led to several developments in information systems applications for radiology services. Because of the radiology department's role and orientation, numerous clinical services and departments now mandate automated and timely reporting of test reports.

Unfortunately, most radiology systems have incorporated functions required for inpatient needs (similar to other departmental systems such as laboratory) but have not fully developed capabilities required for complex ambulatory cases. As ambulatory care growth expands and radiology services reporting becomes a necessity in both hospital-based departments and private physicians' offices, comprehensive information systems dedicated to these needs will no doubt be imperative.

Purpose and Scope of a Radiology Information System

The general purpose and scope of a radiology information system is to allow for on-line ordering and reporting of tests. In addition to these primary functions, a system should also support secondary functions such as maintaining patient logs, test protocols, radiograph locations, and quality control information.

Specifically, at the time of an order request, a system should automatically transfer specific patient demographic, clinical, and financial information already stored in other applications and from a previously assigned patient record number. Additional requests such as surgical procedures ordered, requests referred by a certain physician's office, and so forth, should be available as well.

With a unique patient numbering system, all requests and results can be obtained on-line via a terminal CRT inquiry. This includes verification of the status of tests from any designated CRT, an audit trail of results reporting, film check-out status, and the status of preliminary tests for presurgical cases. Because of the growing importance of point-of-service billing, a system should provide charge generation at the time of examination completion and not at the time of test ordering. A system should also generate a computer-readable medium of services provided by the radiology group(s) for billing purposes.

Although today's information systems will continually evolve to incorporate the demands of outpatients, short-term improvements may well come at the expense of each facility to modify or enhance current system functionality. This may be an easy or difficult task, depending on a system's ability to be enhanced and the commitment of financial and human resources to undertake extensive modifications. Regardless, system applications will need to accommodate as many unique user needs as possible. Of these applications, major needs will include the areas of patient scheduling, tracking the status and reporting of tests, and billing requirements and other administrative functions.

Patient Scheduling

Radiology departments have long been criticized for being inefficient. This has occurred, unfortunately, because scheduling of both inpatients and outpatients is highly complex and because the large numbers of outpatients presenting for examinations are not scheduled. In addition, when patients arrive at a facility for multiple tests, they may be directed to other departments for procedures scheduled to occur at the same appointment time; it may be difficult to locate them at any interval during such testing.

Obviously, the operation of radiology departments is dependent on a systems approach. If patients are not adequately registered and scheduled appropriately by department, examination type, and procedural time(s), they cannot be processed efficiently. Patient scheduling, therefore, is the integral component of a radiology information system. A radiology information system must be highly sophisticated in nature, having the ability to intelligently schedule patients so that they are more evenly distributed throughout the day; be able to follow the patient's course throughout the department; allow system override for emergency or special procedure patients; and accommodate any modifications quickly and without disruption.

At the time of registration, a unique set of data elements should be captured or automatically transferred from other applications. These elements should include the following:

- Patient name
- Address
- Birthdate
- Social security number
- Diagnosis or reason for examination
- Test priority such as today, stat, or preoperative
- Date and time requested
- Name and location of test origin (emergency department, ambulatory surgery, and so forth)
- Patient history number
- Surgery scheduled according to date and time (if applicable)
- Procedures ordered
- Chronic conditions
- Allergies
- Method of patient transportation
- Breakdown of all physicians involved in the care of the patient [for example, ordering, consulting, admitting, and attending physician(s)]

With this basic set of core data elements, sophisticated information management tools can be derived. For instance, once scheduling information is known, it can be manipulated according to predetermined variables such as length of expected procedure time and other patient preparation requirements; availability of procedural rooms by time period; technician staff availability; and other user-defined priorities of tests performed.

Once complete, a system can recommend appointment slots to maximize efficiency. In addition, the information is contained within the system and available at any time for observation of the current status and flow of all patients. With these options, informed decisions regarding staffing allocations and patient service delivery can be enhanced. Although the majority of outpatients are generally considered as "walk-ins" versus appointments, they are scheduled according to the normal appointment process with priority given to the first available time block for any given room.

Test Status, Tracking, and Reporting

A frequent complaint in ancillary service departments is the lack of timely reporting of test results and test tracking (if results are not yet available). Because a schedule-driven system can track the course of a patient's disposition from the scheduled event to bill generation, the patient's profile can be continuously updated and recorded in time intervals.

Although some departments or settings (such as a private physician's office) may not require immediate results reporting, some hospital-based departments (such as the emergency department) will access the system continuously for report updates. In these cases, a system should have unique capabilities that allow immediate access to users via real-time, on-line terminals. These features include the ability to access results immediately by procedural code, patient name, and unit medical record number; the ability to verify uncompleted orders; the ability to perform an audit trail of results reporting; the ability to query patient history information; and the ability to print test results on individual tests as ordered and not simply as a series of tests that were ordered collectively. The emergency department may require that results be maintained on-line for 15 days postdischarge because a certain percentage of patients represent return visits that may result in a hospital admission. Retaining test orders postdischarge for tests required to be completed by the physician is also a frequent request of the emergency department.

Billing Requirements

A schedule-driven information system for radiology also provides accurate reporting for billing purposes. Because all inputs of the system take place at critical points in the patient's care process, a profile of charges is automatically generated for the accounts receivable system. These data also produce the statistical reports reflecting individual service units, scheduling activities, productivity, and facility utilization parameters. Once the registration file is complete (when the patient's examinations are processed and physician-authorized), a system can display the total patient charges plus any outstanding balances. Before the actual entry of the receipt (posting), several system "checks and balances" can be utilized. For instance, underpayments will signal a need for payment justification or explanation, and overpayments will be disallowed. Once totally justified, a printed receipt is available for point-of-service payment, the patient's account reflects the charge/receipt, and the daily journal is updated.

Some facilities may require further specialization of their billing functions. In some situations, a system should allow the user to determine by test, procedure, or service whether to charge at time of results reporting or to charge for tests partially completed with automatic reprinting of orders as necessary. Finally, a system should also specify whether items are patient chargeable or cost center chargeable and should have the capability to specify an update if required.

Administrative Functions

Among the many administrative activities available from a comprehensive information system, daily operational requests and statistical reporting no doubt serve as the most important elements. Of the operational-specific items, a system should have the ability to provide immediate label generation to include unit number, film number, and patient name for radiology film jackets (for filing purposes); the ability to generate an ancillary routing list for radiology patients that includes tests to be performed in other departments; the ability to implement a film checkout system that incorporates date of checkout; due date, requesting party, film destination, film number, and long-term versus short-term storage; and the ability to report past-due films according to user-defined time periods.

In terms of statistical reporting, a system should allow for the purging and reporting of all historical activity data such as room utilization by shift, patient arrival time by room, patient waiting time and equipment usage; the ability to automate listing of services performed according to patient demographic data, including examination type, date of examination, patient type, film file number, and ordering physician; and the ability to generate profiles of examinations according to physician type(s), including attending, ordering, and consulting physician(s).

Conclusion

Information systems for radiology services have yet to be fully extended to the needs of ambulatory care patients. Because the number of outpatients as "walk-ins" creates logistical problems, systems must be capable of immediate patient registration and tracking of a patient's status. In addition, because of its relationship to other departments, on-line, real-time processing and inquiry of test results is not only expected but required in most situations. As radiological technology and testing continues to expand to nontraditional health care settings, systems will also be required to bridge this important information link. Until widespread deployment of these system capabilities occurs, facilities will have to determine whether expanded functionality can be improved through system modifications and at what cost.

Chapter 13

Medical Records

Margret K. Amatayakul

Although computerization of financial and administrative systems has become commonplace at least in larger ambulatory care facilities, computerization of the ambulatory clinical medical record lags behind, just as in hospitals. There are many reasons for automating the clinical medical record. There are also barriers to automation.

Definition of Automated Clinical Medical Record

Before the benefits and constraints of an automated clinical medical record are considered, what constitutes a true automated clinical medical record should be described. There are two components—what is the medical record, and how is it automated?

A medical record is the who, what, when, where, why, and how of patient care. Regardless of the setting in which ambulatory care is provided—solo practice; group practice; health maintenance organization; organized ambulatory care department, emergency department, or special diagnostic/therapeutic department of a hospital; freestanding ambulatory surgery center; or any other applicable location—the care rendered must be carefully documented into a single comprehensive record. Data included are patient and provider demographics, reason for visit, results of physical examination and diagnostic tests, treatment rendered, and plans for followup care.

In 1989, the National Committee on Vital and Health Statistics and the Department of Health and Human Services Interagency Task Force on Uniform Ambulatory Care Data Set published the latest edition of the Uniform Ambulatory Care Data Set. The data set encompasses not only clinical data but financial and administrative data as well.

Other agencies also have defined content standards for ambulatory care medical records. The Joint Commission on Accreditation of Healthcare Organizations (Joint Commission) publishes a standards manual for freestanding ambulatory care facilities (*Ambulatory Health Care Standards Manual*). The medical record standard states that: "The organization maintains a medical record system that permits prompt retrieval of information. Medical records are legible, documented accurately in a timely manner, and readily accessible to health care practitioners." The specific content requirements are listed in figure 13-1.

In its *Accreditation Manual for Hospitals,* the Joint Commission delineates requirements for hospital-sponsored ambulatory care services and emergency services. The medical record content requirements are similar to those for the freestanding ambulatory care facility.

Figure 13-1. Joint Commission Ambulatory Care Medical Record Standards

MR.1.9 A summary list of significant past surgical procedures and past current diagnoses or problems is conspicuously documented in each patient's medical record to facilitate the ongoing provision of effective medical care.

> **MR.1.9.1** The summary list is legibly recorded in the same location in each patient's medical record.
>
> **MR.1.9.2** The summary list does not repeat problems or diagnoses that recur during ongoing treatment.
>
> **MR.1.9.3** The summary list includes, but need not be limited to,
>
>> **MR.1.9.3.1** significant surgical conditions,
>>
>> **MR.1.9.3.2** significant medical conditions,
>>
>> **MR.1.9.3.3** any allergies and untoward reactions to drugs, and
>>
>> **MR.1.9.3.4** currently or recently used medications.

MR.1.10 For each visit, at least the following information is entered in the patient's medical record:

> **MR.1.10.1** Date;
>
> **MR.1.10.2** Department (if the organization is departmentalized);
>
> **MR.1.10.3** Practitioner's name and profession (for example, PT, MD, RN, DDS, DMD);
>
> **MR.1.10.4** Chief complaint or purpose of visit;
>
> **MR.1.10.5** Objective findings;
>
> **MR.1.10.6** Diagnosis or medical impression;
>
> **MR.1.10.7** Studies ordered, such as laboratory or x-ray studies;
>
> **MR.1.10.8** Therapies administered;
>
> **MR.1.10.9** Disposition, recommendations, and instructions to patients; and
>
> **MR.1.10.10** Signatures or initials of practitioners.

Source: Joint Commission on Accreditation of Healthcare Organizations. *Ambulatory Health Care Standards Manual.* Chicago: Joint Commission, 1990.

The Accreditation Association for Ambulatory Health Care (AAAHC) was established in 1979 when the Joint Commission was undergoing organizational changes. The organizations that comprise the AAAHC include the American College Health Association, the American Group Practice Association, the Free Standing Ambulatory Surgical Association, the Group Health Association of America, Inc., the Medical Group Management Association, and the National Association of Community Health Centers, Inc. Standards established by AAAHC for medical records are similar to the Joint Commission standards.

The federal government has established conditions that must be met in order to participate in the Medicare and Medicaid programs. The specific regulations for medical record content are outlined in the *Code of Federal Regulations*. Individual state agencies also specify minimum content requirements for medical records.

The basic data elements and documentation requirements of accrediting and regulatory agencies define the content for the medical record. For the medical record to be automated, all functions related to its creation, use, and storage must be automated. Too often, parts of medical records are generated by computer but are ultimately stored and used in paper form. Although a totally paperless medical record does not happen overnight, it is only through a totally paperless medical record that all benefits of automation can be realized. Figure 13-2 delineates the characteristics of a truly automated medical record.

A truly automated medical record is one that requires no handwritten documentation of clinical data. Intermediary data entry is time-consuming and costly and does not provide the instantaneous access

Figure 13-2. Definition of Automated Medical Record

Data Origination

No handwritten documentation of clinical data.

Input

The same as data origination—no intermediary data entry.

Processing

1. Storage and retrieval of data
2. Conversion of data into information for:

   a. Clinical decision making
   b. Support of facility's business objectives

Output

Easily accessible and readable screens with paper on demand, ensuring privacy and confidentiality.

Storage

1. No paper archiving.
2. Ability to access on demand.

to data that is a hallmark of productivity. A truly automated medical record provides not only storage and retrieval of data but conversion of data (raw facts and figures) into meaningful information (processed data) for clinical decision making. Output is achieved easily and in flexible form. Privacy and confidentiality are ensured. In a paperless system, paper is not archived. Magnetic or optical disk storage media are used with on-line, real-time access capabilities.

Benefits of an Automated Ambulatory Clinical Medical Record

The primary reason for an automated ambulatory clinical medical record is improved productivity of physicians and their support staffs. Efficient use of time is the measure of productivity. The automated clinical medical record contributes to efficient use of time in several ways.

First, the automated clinical medical record contributes to efficiency because it is accessible. There is virtually no time required to wait for a record to be retrieved from a file, and there is virtually no chance for a lost or temporarily misplaced record. Even if two staff members must access a record at one time, both can do so on-line, simultaneously. When a paper record cannot be found on a day a patient is scheduled for an appointment, it can disrupt the entire day's schedule. Telephone inquiries, requests for prescription renewals, and so forth often require review of the patient's record. The time required to pull and replace the record can take longer than the actual review. With an automated system, the patient record can be retrieved without leaving one's desk. The same principle holds true for laboratory technicians who need to review prior test results, office personnel who need patient demographics, and nurses who handle questions regarding immunization information or dates of past events.

The second way the automated clinical medical record can improve productivity is through improved record review capabilities. Although all documentation may be input into an automated medical record, it is not necessary to review the entire set of documentation to review specific pieces of data, as is true for paper medical records. Critical data points such as medications, vital signs, test results, and other structured data (for example, problems, allergies, and drug reactions) can be isolated for review. The data can be displayed in flowcharts or in graphic format to help spot trends. Information that can be structured can be displayed in a consistent and user-definable format to facilitate review. Data that cannot be structured, such as encounter notes, can be keyed to a structured problem list to facilitate retrieval. Hospital-generated information can also be stored in the automated record system and segregated upon retrieval if desired. Isolating similar information in easy-to-retrieve locations reduces record review time.

Data base review for clinical research, quality assurance, and utilization management is also enhanced with an automated clinical medical record. An automated data base can be searched in minutes or hours to find information that would take days or weeks to assemble from paper records. The computer is good at tracking subtle trends. It can easily offer suggestions for a patient's treatment from information it holds about hundreds of similar cases. In some cases, certain searches would not even have been attempted in a paper environment because the effort required was too great. This is especially true in the case of tasks such as practice marketing and modeling activities.

A fully automated clinical medical record system containing these features can potentially cut record review times by 50 percent or more. To the physician seeing 20 to 30 patients per day, this could mean 30 to 60 minutes of additional time each day. In a year, this can amount to several days or weeks of time. The value of this time can be measured by factoring in the incremental profit margin rates of the physician's practice.

Less tangible than improved productivity, but no less important, are benefits accrued to patients. Patients benefit from any system that has the potential to improve the physician's working conditions. An automated medical record system provides the physician greater amounts of information that can be dealt with quickly and efficiently. A properly designed system provides the physician with a tool to aid in delivery of the best possible quality of care. It frees the physician to spend more time listening to, examining, instructing, and prescribing for the patient. Not only does this ensure high-quality care, but it benefits practice building as well. Many market studies show that the primary reason a patient changes physicians is because the physician is perceived as not paying enough attention to the patient. Patients are loyal to their physicians and make referrals on their behalf when they perceive that they are getting attention.

In the event that a medical record must be reviewed by another physician, consultant, auditor, or attorney, the automated medical record is neat and legible.

Barriers to Automating the Medical Record

Although the benefits of an automated clinical medical record are clear, it has taken many years of technological advances to approach the truly automated clinical medical record. The wide gap between paper and paperless has been due to the wide gap between medical communication and computer technology. This gap comes in many forms.

One of the most difficult barriers to automation of the medical record is the man–machine interface. Inputting data by keyboard or even touch screens, light pens, optical character recognition, bar coding, and point-and-click mouse systems has been less than satisfactory. An automated medical record system must not force physicians to change their current practices (unless they wish to, in which case the system must be flexible enough to do so). Digital dictation and voice recognition systems are just now being developed to bridge the gap between the person and the computer for entry of data. Until voice recognition systems can reliably capture the full range of vocabulary used by the medical profession at normal speaking rates, data entry will remain the most significant barrier to automation of the medical record.

Barriers other than hardware also relate to input. Many existing systems have a highly structured format and require standardized terminology. Entering data into a structured format with standard terms can be very time-consuming and frustrating. It has not been until very recently that the sciences of text processing and medical informatics have come into being. Computers can deal with numeric data but cannot understand nonnumeric information. Medical terms are linguistic representations of concepts, not symbols, and thus are incompatible with computer technology. In the laboratories of some physicians and at the National Library of Medicine, work is being conducted on establishing a coded comprehensive medical nomenclature. Such research will assist in manipulating text data.

Some of the same barriers that exist for input also exist for output. Retrieval of data from an automated medical record must be able to be performed in English with a minimum amount of structured elements that must be responded to. Output should be in a readable form. Output from many systems has been cryptic at best. Both screen display and paper output should be accommodated easily.

Security, confidentiality, privacy, admissibility, and safety are also issues that must be resolved in an automated clinical medical record system.

Many health care providers are uncomfortable with computer storage of medical records. Paper medical records are much more prone to loss, but most providers have not yet accepted the totally paperless medical record concept, even though backup—which never existed in a paper system—can be performed easily and economically.

Aside from personal preference, admissibility of computerized medical records is the most significant factor to consider. The courts have addressed the issue of computer-stored records for at least a decade, and they have not found magnetic storage to be a stumbling block. An expert in the field notes that "optical disks are nonerasable and are actually a more trustworthy medium than magnetic disk or tape. . . . In time, optical will enjoy legal parity in case law with microfilm. It already has that parity in statutory law."

The medium used to store records is not the issue in legal cases; how the records are stored and used is much more important. Courts have used three criteria in deciding whether to admit computer-stored records: the safeguards that are in place to ensure accuracy, the presumption of reliability through regular business use of the system, and the manner in which the system is secured.

Factors to consider in developing data accuracy controls include the purpose of the controls, identification of areas within a computerized medical record where error can occur, and decisions about correction of errors. Controls must detect the existence of an error, must locate the error (or all possible points of error), and must provide for the correction of the error. Validity and reasonableness checking can be programmed into a medical record system to aid in detection of errors. It should be remembered that data can be more accurate in a computer system because of the ability to program decision pathways that must be completed; and inaccurate data are more apparent in a computer system than in a manual system, although possibly no more prevalent because error detection programs apply to all data.

When the regular business use of computerized medical records comes under legal scrutiny, the manner in which the records are compiled and used is evaluated. It is generally accepted that the use of passwords, keys, and so forth are equivalent to a signature for authentication purposes. The degree of care taken in securing these alternative forms of authentication, however, may have to be proved. Record linkage also may cause some legal confusion. Issues of who owns the medical record and who is responsible for the accuracy of the data and security of the system are important to clarify.

Data security refers to two issues: data loss and data misuse. *Data loss* refers to the actual physical loss of data from the computer or from off-line storage via theft, natural disaster, or other power failure. Specific protections, backup systems, maintenance procedures, and recovery procedures must be in place. Controls for *data misuse* must exist over access to the system's inputs and outputs to ensure that patients' privacy is not violated and that data are maintained confidentially. Security systems must be in place that allow only authorized users to access or change medical record content.

When automation of the medical record encompasses medical decision making, the extent of the system that is admissible may come under question. Although the Food and Drug Administration has ruled that computer systems are not medical devices, the area is still somewhat grey with respect to liability. Strict protocols should be established when artificial intelligence, or expert systems, are included in the automated medical record.

Automated Medical Record Systems

Several ambulatory care organizations have been instrumental in developing ambulatory medical record systems. The most widely used or most developed are COSTAR (Computer Stored Ambulatory Record), RMRS (Regenstrief Medical Record System), STOR (Summary Time Oriented Record), and TMR (The Medical Record).

The COSTAR system is comprised of six modules. The security and integrity module provides for user identification and access. The registration module allows for the entry, service, and modification of the patient registration data. A scheduling module supports an appointment system. The medical record module processes the medical data. Many systems in place still use an encounter form as a source document for this purpose. There are also a billing and accounts receivable module and a management reporting module. COSTAR includes a Medical Query Language (MQL), which permits users with no programming background to search the data base for ad hoc information needs.

Bibliography

Amatayakul, M. K. Automating the medical record. Presentation at HIMSS Greater Chicago chapter, Sept. 29, 1988.

Cerne, F. Optical disk technology: going paperless. *Hospitals* 62(10):94–95, May 20, 1988.

Feste, L. K. *Ambulatory Care Documentation.* Chicago: American Medical Record Association, 1989.

Gabrieli, E. R., and Murphy, G. Computerized medical records. *Journal of the American Medical Record Association,* vol. 61, Jan. 1990.

Gardner, E. Automated medical chart becoming a priority. *Modern Healthcare* 18(35):29–52, Sept. 2, 1988.

Groom, D. Automation of the medical chart. *Computers in Healthcare* 8(14):22–28, Dec. 1987.

Huffman, E. K. Medical record management. In: Finnegan, R. M., and Amatayakul, M. K., editors. *Information Systems in Health Care.* 9th ed. Berwyn, IL: Physicians' Record Company, 1990.

Joint Commission on Accreditation of Healthcare Organizations. Medical records. *Ambulatory Health Care Standards Manual.* Chicago: Joint Commission, 1990, pp. 15–17.

McKnight, W. G. Voice recognition technology. *Journal of the American Medical Record Association* 58(12):28–29, Dec. 1987.

National Committee on Vital and Health Statistics Subcommittee on Ambulatory Care Statistics and the Interagency Task Force on the Uniform Ambulatory Care Data Set, *Uniform Ambulatory Care Data Set,* June 1989.

Rutherford, W. E. Automating the clinical record. *Computers in Healthcare* 8(14):50–54, Dec. 1987.

Chapter 14

Clinical Laboratories

Raymond D. Aller, M.D.

Many of the information processing requirements of clinical laboratories in the ambulatory setting are similar to those for laboratories serving inpatients;[1-3] however, some ambulatory care laboratories, such as regional blood banks, have highly specialized needs.[4] Within ambulatory medicine, varying organizational structures lead to different system requirements. This chapter briefly summarizes the unique requirements of clinical laboratories in the ambulatory care setting, and reviews how one laboratory serving several hundred independent practitioners has dealt with these issues.

The ambulatory care laboratory (clinic laboratory) serving a closed panel of physicians (for example, a large multispecialty group practice) is subject to quite different demands and requirements than a laboratory serving large numbers of independent practitioners and clinics. Typically, a group practice will have assigned permanent patient numbers to each patient, and billing information will have been collected when the patient was first seen at the group practice. In a group practice situation, orders for future laboratory tests must be queued, but a mechanism must exist for order cancellation when the patient has not appeared within a few days of the scheduled test. Rapid turnaround time is often required, because a patient may go to the laboratory shortly before a scheduled physician appointment, with the physician counting on laboratory results for immediate patient management. Because a common patient chart is shared by all practitioners, agreement is reached on the "optimal" format for reporting. Longitudinal, cumulative patient reports are relatively straightforward to produce in such a setting because of the permanent patient number, although the format and scheduling required for these reports differs from a typical inpatient cumulative report. In most respects, the clinic laboratory shares characteristics with a hospital laboratory. Therefore, it is not surprising that some laboratory information systems designed for hospitals (inpatient and outpatient services) have worked well in group practice laboratories.

An entirely different situation exists for the independent laboratory. Such laboratories face challenges not encountered elsewhere in laboratory medicine, and they require specially designed software packages or extensive modifications in systems designed for hospital laboratories. These challenges include:

- Patient identification/record linkage
- Scheduling/tracking of test orders and specimens
- Effects of prolonged or suboptimal specimen transport
- Conflicting demands for test profiles and report formats
- Printing and inquiry of reports to remote locations
- An intensely competitive environment
- Complex billing requirements

Patient Identification and Record Linkage

Most specimens are submitted to independent laboratories without a permanent, numeric patient identifier. This poses no problem for the laboratory that restricts itself to performing chemistry panels and urinalysis, but may adversely affect patient care in cytopathology, surgical pathology, blood banking, immunology (particularly tumor markers), and hematology. Larger clients, who maintain their own permanent chart number, can be encouraged to submit this number, but if the patient sees another physician, the record will not be collated. Some laboratories have encouraged the use of the social security number. Despite transcription errors commonly occurring with a nine-digit number, patients who may not have a social security number, and patients who remember the number incorrectly, this is probably the easiest method for record linkage today. An alternative is to link patients on the basis of name and birthdate (name, or name and age, alone are *not* adequate); using equivalency tables for first names (for example, Beth, Liz, and Betty match with Elizabeth), improves retrieval rates. A methodology with superior performance in tracking cytological histories is used by Dr. George Wied's department at the University of Chicago: women are indexed under their mother's maiden name and their own birthdate. In any case, manual intervention is usually required to evaluate whether a proposed match or linkage is appropriate. Once a reliable linkage has been established, computers have valuable capabilities in producing cumulative reports of numerical values, and historical searches of diagnostic histories in blood banks, hematology, cytopathology, and surgical pathology.

Scheduling and Tracking of Test Orders and Specimens

Once a specimen has left the client's office, the laboratory assumes responsibility for it. Using devices such as portable bar-code scanners, laboratories are beginning to implement systems recording specimen pickup and tracking of transport. Such technology has already proved extremely worthwhile for in-laboratory specimen handling.[5]

The client typically indicates test orders on a paper requisition or log sheet. When special panels have been devised for a physician's use, these order codes, together with the client number, should be preprinted onto the requisition.

Effects of Prolonged or Suboptimal Specimen Transport

When patient specimens are traveling from long distances to reach the laboratory, or are collected in the physician's office early in the day but not picked up by the laboratory until evening, several artifacts appear that are uncommon in a hospital setting. For this reason, it is desirable for the information system to be able to track collection time, pickup time, time of receipt in the central laboratory, and time of spindown/aliquotting. Armed with a sheet of cases all showing elevated levels of potassium and abnormal lactic dehydrogenase, closely correlated with prolonged delays between collection and aliquotting, it may become easier to convince the physician and his or her office staff to spin and separate specimens.

Conflicting Demands for Test Profiles and Report Formats

Experience has shown that every physician has a different idea about which tests are wanted and how they should be arranged on the report form. The information system should permit establishing, and customizing for each client, special test panels, automatic followup testing rules, telephone reporting rules, printed report layouts, and the like. Earlier generations of software required prohibitively expensive custom reprogramming to accomplish this; more recent systems put these capabilities into a series of tables under user control.

Printing and Inquiry of Reports to Remote Locations

The wide geographic area covered by the typical independent laboratory is served more effectively by electronically transmitting completed

reports to outlying clients or to branch laboratories in the client's community. A reliable telephone system, coupled with error-correcting modems,
has made this quite inexpensive and practical. However, special programming is required within the information system to effectively control the
modems, and to automatically diagnose the wide variety of "trance states"
that remote printers seem to enter. Troubleshooting of remote printers has
been further simplified by the recent introduction (by at least three vendors) of modem-printer packages. A more complex approach permits the
client site to dial into the laboratory computer and inquire about test status and previous results, as well as print the current results.

Intensely Competitive Environment

One of the most striking differences between many hospital laboratories
and the typical independent laboratory is the attitude toward customer
concerns and complaints. The hospital laboratory has a guaranteed exclu-
sive to serve those hospital inpatients – unless there is a severe, chronic
failure to provide service. In the independent laboratory, there is a general
realization that a seemingly minor service problem or perceived lack of
responsiveness may lead clients to send their work to one of the three or
four other laboratories vying for their business. Therefore, a highly reliable reporting system is essential for independent laboratories. At the same
time, the laboratory is constantly upgrading its services to gain a competitive advantage with features such as interpretive reporting, graphic output, and more sensitive and specific analytic technology. All of these
require increasingly sophisticated laboratory information systems.

Complex Billing Requirements

In some settings, there may be as many ways of billing a test as the laboratory has clients! The increasing complexity of Medicare billing is combined with HMO rules, capitation plans, special discount arrangements,
and even "loss leaders." Charges differ depending on whether the patient
pays at the time of specimen collection or must be billed. Tests performed
on the weekend may be more costly than routinely performed tests during the week. With this complexity, a good independent laboratory billing system may be every bit as complex as the other modules of the
laboratory information system combined.

An Application Case Study

Having described the challenges facing the implementation of information systems in independent laboratories, this chapter will conclude by

describing the system being used in one such laboratory in California. The laboratory serves about 300 physicians in a 125-mile radius, processes 700 specimens per day, and employs 85 full-time-equivalent staff. In addition to three drawing stations, the laboratory has two "stat" laboratories in cities 70 and 120 miles, respectively, from the main laboratory. Laboratory specimen processing and reporting is facilitated by a software package licensed from a popular laboratory information system (LIS) vendor, with modifications by laboratory staff to provide some of the special functions mentioned in this chapter. The laboratory has written special software to drive modems for remote transmittal of reports, and it currently transmits reports several times each day to about 20 different locations, using error-correcting modems. "Leased" lines with multiplexors are used to connect terminals and printers in its stat laboratories to the main computer. In addition, these leased lines are used to position a modem closer to some remote clients, reducing the long-distance charges that would otherwise be incurred.

Computer hardware, like any electric device, will occasionally fail. Unfortunately, the competitive marketplace does not tolerate even a temporary failure of the laboratory computer—clients want the report *now*. Therefore, a recent (and near-disastrous) three-day downtime because of undiagnosable hardware ills precipitated the decision to move to a redundant hardware configuration, so that even a major hardware failure would require no more than a few minutes of system unavailability. Some vendors base all their systems on such hardware; others have redundancy available as an option for those settings where it is particularly required.

The information system has made it possible for the laboratory to provide other services as well, which would have been impossible in a manual setting. These include an automatic interpretive comment with all hepatitis serology panels, a "reflexive" followup testing panel (certain abnormalities on the chemistry panel or complete blood count will generate further diagnostic tests), and graphical/trend reports for tumor market assays. Each client has its own panels and receives customized report formats.

The laboratory information system is linked to a separate billing computer, running software from a different vendor. Special billing rules have been built into both systems—for example, certain clients are always "bill patient," so that the laboratory system will not accept a "bill client" indication.

Information systems have been vital to the survival and growth of this independent laboratory. In other areas of ambulatory medicine, it may be possible to function adequately without computer support, but a fully functional and flexible computer system is the standard of practice and the key to survival in the independent laboratory arena.

Conclusion

A well-implemented laboratory information system can provide a competitive edge for independent laboratories. Laboratory information systems can produce statistical reports and historical searches of diagnostic histories, track collection and pickup times for specimens, customize test report formats, print and permit inquiry of reports to remote locations, and handle complex billing requirements.

References

1. Elevitch, F. R., and Aller, R. D. *The ABCs of LIS*. Revised ed. Chicago: ASCP Press, 1989.

2. Aller, R. D., and Elevitch, F. R. Symposium on computers in the clinical laboratory. *Clinics in Laboratory Medicine* 3(1):1–254, Mar. 1983.

3. Weilert, M., Aller, R. D., and Pasia, O. G. Clinical laboratory information systems survey. *CAP TODAY* 3(11):20–37, Nov. 1989.

4. Aller, R. D., Weilert, M., and Pasia, O. G. Blood bank information systems. *CAP TODAY* 3(10):52–58, Oct. 1989.

5. Tilzer, L., and Jones, R. W. Use of barcode labels on collection tubes for specimen management in the clinical laboratory. *Archives of Pathology and Laboratory Medicine* 112(12):1200–02, Dec. 1988.

Chapter 15

Multiple Freestanding Facilities

Margaret D. Sabin and Thomas A. Stocker

This chapter attempts to describe some of the key information aspects of multiple freestanding ambulatory medical centers. Many of the key points for this chapter have come from the experience of the Medical Centers of Colorado network, which is located in metropolitan Denver and is affiliated with Lutheran Medical Center. However, the chapter is presented in fairly generic form. Given the dynamic and highly fragmented field of outpatient care, the experience of one provider is just that: the experience of *one* provider. Although it is too early to evaluate the experience of the Medical Centers of Colorado, many important points can be gleaned from its system selection and implementation process. The Medical Centers of Colorado network is comprised of seven sites located to provide geographic coverage for the Denver metropolitan area. Five of these sites are running on the Annson Response System, with additional sites scheduled for implementation in 1990.

In a growing number of ambulatory care situations, information systems are becoming critical to the strategic prospects of the entire organization. The administrator is likely to spend an increasing amount of time thinking about problems or opportunities resulting from the information systems operation. In these settings, as this chapter explores, the administrator is concerned about information systems and their role in product development, information availability, and linkage to affiliated enterprises such as host hospitals.

State of the Art of Outpatient Information Systems

In the past two decades, much attention has been focused on the development of functionally rich inpatient hospital information systems.

This is particularly true among the vendor community, which has made impressive products available to hospitals. Recently, these vendors have begun to develop approaches to incorporate outpatient information, such as coding and abstracting of Medicare outpatient surgery episodes, but these efforts remain predominantly hospital-based. A problem stems from hospital perception that virtually all of the information systems development resources should be allocated toward the support of traditional hospital applications. A recent study by McManis and Associates suggests that this perception is incongruent with future health care provider service trends. The study contends that hospital-based activity will decline dramatically by the year 2000, and that outpatient services, especially those performed in freestanding ambulatory care centers, will subsequently increase. Thus, resources budgeted toward information systems development will be shifted over time toward outpatient applications systems.

Components of freestanding ambulatory care information systems have evolved over the past five years. Fairly impressive general financial systems that process general ledger, payroll, and accounts payable are in place. Other systems that can perform some scheduling functions and basic quality assurance/review are available as well. General patient accounting/billing systems are common—but typically dysfunctional as they attempt to retrofit individual-practice billing systems to handle quantities of transactions inappropriate to high-volume ambulatory care centers. Most of these systems are standalone and are not consistently maintained. Currently, these systems interface with hospital information systems poorly, or not at all. For many health care provider networks, this disjointed approach could contribute to potentially disastrous business practices.

Issues Affecting Ambulatory Information Systems

The move to ambulatory care has progressed steadily over the past 10 to 15 years, bringing a number of new challenges and requirements to information systems. During the past 5 to 10 years, hospitals have reorganized into corporate entities, which has provided a framework for multiple business entities. It is within the for-profit arms of these corporate entities that freestanding ambulatory care centers (ACCs) generally reside. Corporate entities may have singular or dual objectives for establishing these entities, including attaining standalone profitability or facilitating referrals to the host hospital or occupational medicine network. All of the objectives, and the priority of these objectives, affect the system selection process.

Front-door feeder systems are particularly well positioned for competitive advantages because they draw from a larger geographic area than that of a standalone hospital. These entities are therefore highly in need of comprehensive automated systems. Access to clinical and financial information is a critical bargaining point for employers that are individually and collectively attempting to decrease their employee health costs through designated-provider affiliations.

The overriding issue affecting information systems design within the freestanding ambulatory care center is how integrated the center will be in the context of a provider network. Because of geographic proximity and physician participation, freestanding ambulatory care centers are natural partners to host hospitals eager to position themselves for favorable contract negotiations. Assuming a relationship between the ambulatory care centers and host hospital that is much more integrated, the following issues are those that will have a significant impact on information systems:

- *A centralized, master patient index accessible from any mode of the provider network.* This capability would allow the network to better track patient encounters as demanded by third-party payers, particularly related to the growing workers' compensation business.
- *Enhanced nursing care provider functionality.* Quality improvement and care provider productivity could be prospectively achieved through successful implementation of applications such as on-line charting.
- *High-speed data communications.* The most logical step beyond a centralized master patient index on-line charting is the concept of the centralized or "paperless" medical record. Such applications require tremendous amounts of data storage and, therefore, very high communications speeds to retrieve data.
- *A flexible, integrated clinical/financial data base.* The provider network needs immediate access to integrated information to compete for third-party payer contracts and to prepare proactively for Medicare reimbursement methodology to evolve, that is, toward pending prospective systems or even capitation. This might also allow tracing of service lines and a patient's entire episode of illness. As the field increasingly faces declining operating margins, detailed data on costs and service utilization are necessary.
- *Information systems planning.* Experts freely acknowledge that the health care industry will experience dynamic changes for the foreseeable future. Outpatient care provision is particularly unpredictable, because it is within ambulatory care that major growth of services is contemplated. Reimbursement methodology, technology improvements, and a shift of population ages are all examples of variables that will influence how health care provider networks conduct their business. Because of the self-evident need to plan for flexible information systems, the following planning issues are especially relevant:
  - *Incorporation of benefits of hospital sophistication.* Hospitals generally do a good job in processing large quantities of transactions, whether

they are orders, bills, or paychecks. Within the concept of a provider network, it is desirable to exploit some of this experience to benefit the freestanding ambulatory care center. This is especially true within information systems applications that process relevant information such as medical records. The first step in achieving a centralized master patient index, for example, would be to work with the hospital staff to formulate standard forms and indexing methodology.

– *Development of a minimum standard clinical/financial data set.* To support the objective of tracking patient encounters throughout the entire health care provider network, a minimum standard data set is indicated. The data set would provide a foundation for clinical, operational, and strategic decision making by giving clinical/financial information in such a manner so that management of the "bottom line" is a daily focus. Considerable planning and negotiating would be needed to ensure that all providers within the network participate in creating and maintaining this single data base, updating it every time a patient is encountered.

– *Development of nationally accepted ambulatory data standards.* One of the factors confounding growth in the availability and sophistication of outpatient data systems is the lack of a uniform, nationally accepted ambulatory data set (as discussed in chapter 8). This issue, combined with the uncertainty over the specific composition of the ambulatory payment system, makes vendors reluctant to invest system development efforts in a changing situation. However, progress is being made in this area at the federal level.

Network Information Needs

Information needs form various levels in the freestanding, hospital-affiliated entities. At the most basic level, and probably the key impetus for automation, would be requirements of third-party billing. The "cash and carry" business is eroding as more insurance plans, HMOs, PPOs, and employer-directed plans control the market. Information needs form a pyramid with financial packages at the base level; clinical, financial, and demographic data at the next level; physician production patterns at the next level; and other market information and general planning information at the top level. The base-level financial package includes components for insurance billing, general ledger, and accounts payable. Most packages currently on the market meet this basic level of need.

The second tier of information includes patient clinical and demographic information and should pull from the billing document and the medical record, if it is automated. This tier enables the group administrator to analyze the specifics of the customer base. Frequently, this is an area of analysis that group administrators have little time to attend to. As the trend toward hospital affiliation continues, this area will grow in importance as the expectations of the group administrator shift from standalone, bottom-line performance to integration into a larger health care system.

Although the third area, that of physician production and performance, is not listed as a top-priority area, it is attended to fairly well by most group packages. Compensation arrangements for the group probably include incentive compensation of physicians on a production basis.

It is extremely important to recognize that these capabilities may shift in terms of their importance to the provider. Many who choose a package for its billing module assume that the other capabilities are either there or can be developed by the manufacturer. This is a potentially dangerous assumption. Many of the smaller software companies that initially produce these products are acquired by larger entities interested in the original company for cash. Their commitment to the client in terms of system updating and development may not be the same as the stated commitment of the original company.

Getting Started

A key consideration in the introduction of automation to a multisite ambulatory network is the actual setup. Some entities opt to use a system that can be started as an offsite, batch-processing network, whereas others look for direct access via terminals in the centers. In the latter approach, the up-front expense would be decreased. There are many systems on the market that can be purchased in this mode and can be converted to onsite status down the line. However, institutional goals and the health care environment (particularly for data processing) are subject to change. Selecting a system that is flexible enough to accommodate change is prudent.

Frequently, the team completing the plan for system selection includes the group practice administrator, the group medical director, the individual at the host hospital with umbrella responsibility over the ACC, and the information systems director from the host hospital. An area that never gets enough consideration is the impact of a system on ongoing operating costs of the entity and the revenue enhancement that can be expected to accrue from system implementation. In the current environment, it is difficult to cost-justify these systems, particularly on a standalone basis. Again, corporate goals must enter into this analysis because the system may require support on the up-front system acquisition and possibly for ongoing operating costs.

The margin in ambulatory care, particularly the ACC environment, is relatively slim and not entirely immune to erosion. If the margin is currently at an average of $10 per patient visit, the financial drain of on-going support of an automated system may decrease this margin to $6 or $7 per patient. Too often, group practice administrators assume huge increases in insurance patients, but many markets are quickly becoming saturated with options for outpatient care, and huge increases in patients may not be possible. Instead, it may ensure that the ACC will keep its current patient load and keep up with the competition.

The up-front support of the group practice physicians is critical to the success of the system. The support of these individuals cannot be undervalued, particularly if the acquisition and ongoing operating costs of the system are to be counted against the cost structure of the individual ACCs. Communication regarding the goals for the system and reasonably achievable benefits will produce a feeling of being part of the decision and, thus, potential support for the system.

Conclusion

Making a decision regarding network automation in the current environment is much more difficult than making an automation decision for the relatively stable inpatient environment. On the inpatient side, there is a nationally accepted uniform inpatient data set; as mentioned previously, this does not exist on the outpatient side. On the inpatient side, reimbursement changed seven years ago, and vendors responded with systems that could handle a diagnosis related group type of reimbursement system. Reimbursement for outpatient services remains in a state of flux, and there are almost as many methods of reimbursement as there are third-party payers. Yet, ACCs need to respond to an increasingly competitive, saturated market and may not be able to afford the luxury of waiting for data standardization to bring about more flexible systems. In this environment, caution, cynicism (particularly regarding vendors' promises), communication (particularly with key physicians), and flexibility are all necessary components of successful system implementation. Making a decision that will gain or at least protect the market share of an ACC will ensure its continued viability into an era when the "perfect" ambulatory information system is created.

Chapter 16

Referral Management Systems

Jill Crowell

Renewed emphasis on cost and quality has led to the use of referral management systems as a multipurpose tool in ambulatory care settings. This chapter describes why referral management systems are needed, how they work, and how they can be applied in utilization review/quality assurance, operations, and budgeting and cost management.

Managing for Cost and Quality

A brief mention of the factors that have led to increased outpatient utilization and costs is helpful in understanding the environment in which referral management systems operate. Increased outpatient utilization and costs are, among other things, attributed to more use of high technology in outpatient settings, the less controlled environment of outpatient care where services are more patient-initiated, and the lack of analytic and control methodologies for outpatient care. Several other factors have affected outpatient care similar to the way they have influenced inpatient care. Lower reimbursement levels, tougher utilization review including more stringent review of diagnostic tests, increased case management, and more direct contracting with providers and physicians who meet cost-conscious standards have begun to affect outpatient care delivery and will continue to do so.

Outpatient services will also see greater scrutiny of service quality brought about on the inpatient side by DRGs and other cost-management methodologies. Third-party payers and businesses are looking for credible systems that will assess the quality of care aspects of prepaid health plans. (This issue was covered in *Healthcare Financial News*, May 15, 1988, p. 9.)

Hospitals, clinics, and individual practitioners must be prepared not only to manage for cost and quality but also to provide utilization and service quality data for both inpatient and outpatient settings. Automated referral management systems are increasingly being viewed as tools to support cost and quality management.

What Are Referral Management Systems?

Referral management systems (RMS) are designed to support organizations where operations, at least in part, reflect the following assumptions:

- Cost containment will be most effective where services are preauthorized.
- Preauthorization of services provides a mechanism for defining and managing aspects of service quality.
- Managing service cost and quality requires the availability of timely information regarding what services are provided to whom, by whom, for what purposes, at what cost, and with what results.

Thus, in their current manifestation, referral management systems are viewed largely as tools for managed care settings.

As with other management control mechanisms, preauthorizing services raises operational issues of sometimes astounding complexity. In preparation for a new referral management system, the business office staff of a large long-standing and successful managed care organization identified the following referral-related problems—problems strikingly familiar to others who work in managed care settings:

- The care prescribed is not necessarily obtained.
- We don't know if we've exceeded referral time or how to manage it better.
- We don't know who is responsible for monitoring care when a patient is sent outside for care as a result of internal backlogs.
- We don't know when a followup referral is needed.
- We don't know when a patient has used a referral.
- We don't know if and when patients should return to us after an external referral.
- We can't track internal referrals, self-referrals, or external inpatient referrals.
- We don't have a consistent method for knowing if and when coverage has cleared.
- Physicians refer without a referral form; we can't track these referrals.
- We don't have referral summary information on a weekly basis to identify and solve problems.

Referral management systems are designed to address these and similar problems. Simply stated, RMS provide automated tools for pre-authorizing services and subsequently validating claims received against authorized referrals. They work in much the same way as purchase-order systems, where expenditures are authorized and expenses estimated before the expenditures actually occur.

Although straightforward in concept, the referral management process is one of considerable complexity, requiring access to updating and retrieval of information from a wide array of patient, provider, coverage, claims, clinical, and RMS operations files. The RMS process is described below not in its detail and complexity but in high-level summary. The intent is to provide a framework for later discussion of RMS benefits and reports.

How Referral Management Systems Work

Referral management systems can track and process internal, external, emergency, and self-referrals for both inpatient and outpatient services. Referral management systems are not all the same, of course. Generally speaking, however, and using an external referral to illustrate, the referral management process works in the following way:

- *Step 1.* The referring practitioner's office forwards a completed external referral request form to the referral authorization office.
- *Step 2.* A referral authorization staff person reviews the request for completeness, accuracy, and compliance with medical and other appropriate protocols.
- *Step 3.* If the referral request meets completion, accuracy, and compliance requirements, the request is entered on-line. Otherwise, action is taken to resolve the request's deficiencies.
- *Step 4.* Once the referral request data are entered into the system, the system inquires of the membership and benefits data bases to determine the patient's eligibility for the requested service(s).
  - If the patient is eligible for the requested service(s), the system produces a referral authorization document, which is sent to the patient and the provider/practitioner to whom the patient is referred. The authorization document identifies the authorized service(s) and the time frames in which the service(s) is to be delivered. At this time, the system can also generate a cost estimate for the referred service(s).
  - If the patient is not eligible for the requested service(s), the system prints a recommendation for a noncovered service document. This document is sent to the patient and the provider/practitioner to whom the patient is recommended for care. This document clarifies that the patient is being recommended for specific care but that the care will not be paid for by the referring organization.

- *Step 5.* Once claims for services are logged into the claims-processing system, they are validated against RMS preauthorization records. (Claims are, of course, also validated against other files such as patient utilization history, provider files, and so forth.) Claims not within the authorized scope of care (that is, type and amount of service, specific provider/practitioner, dates of care, and so forth) are suspended for manual review and resolution. Otherwise, the claim is flagged by RMS as ready for further processing.

Throughout this process, historical records are created, producing the data bases from which management reports are produced and data are accessed for the cost and quality management processes. For example, budget and location data are collected for the referring practitioner, services and referrals are identified by type, referral status (such as completed or deleted) is updated, and suspended claims are flagged. Reports are generated on a daily, weekly, or monthly basis, depending on the nature of and purpose for which a report is produced. Examples of reports would include deleted referrals, incomplete referrals, inpatient census by facility, referring practitioner activity, monthly referral activity by budget center, referrals to specialty centers, referral activity by diagnosis, emergency referrals, self-referrals, and so forth, all of which can be cross-referenced with other variables or limited to reflect the information of interest. The following examples show how these reports can be used to identify problems and spot trends:

1. Patterns in external referrals might identify areas for training, needs for new technology or new services, or needs for changes in coverage.
2. Practitioner referral activity might be used for annual practitioner reviews or for taking action to prevent unnecessary referrals.
3. Wait time reports might identify backlogged areas or service quality issues.
4. Trends in referrals to ancillary services by diagnosis might identify needs for service protocol development.

Figures 16-1 to 16-3 identify additional selected ways in which referral management systems are used in utilization review/quality assurance, budget/financial, and cost management and operations. (It is important to note that because referral management systems work in conjunction with claims-processing systems, some RMS benefits derive from this relationship rather than from the RMS system alone.)

Conclusion

Certain tools provided by some referral management systems are at a level of sophistication most organizations are not prepared to use. For example, some referral management systems can, in varying degrees, automate in the preauthorization process the use of service protocols for cost and quality management. To use this feature, however, the organization needs to have a developed set of service protocols to automate. Most organizations do not have such protocols. In the same way, using the cost-estimating feature of a referral management system requires that an organization have manual cost-estimating methods such that they can be automated. In many respects, then, referral management systems represent a future for managing cost and quality rather than today's reality.

Figure 16-1. RMS Uses in Utilization Review/Quality Assurance

1. Monitor consumer care by external providers:
   —Ensure that patients are seen in a timely fashion (check wait times; see that patients use referrals).
   —Ensure that followup care is completed in accordance with protocols (give tickler list to physicians; ensure that the provider seen is the provider referred to).
   —Stop referrals that have expired or are no longer covered (that is, stop liability).
2. Compare rates of referrals among physicians to internal and external specialties.
3. Monitor trends in referral rates over time.
4. Monitor profiles of physician referral patterns.
5. Monitor cost and utilization profiles for members by age, sex, family, employer type, and zip codes.
6. Identify problems in care patterns (underutilization or overutilization of services, emergency referral and self-referral abuse).
7. Identify referral authorizations that are within specific time periods of expiration (such as one week, two weeks). (Practitioners can authorize extensions of the time period for the referral.)

Source: Modified from documents produced at Group Health Cooperative of Puget Sound, Seattle, Washington.

Figure 16-2. RMS Uses in Operations

1. Achieve operational efficiencies through integration of automated functions into day-to-day functions.
2. Gain rapid access to needed information (such as eligibility, benefits) for daily tasks while minimizing reliance on paper files.
3. Get point-of-referral patient information on co-pays and service limits.
4. Improve public relations through rapid access to information in response to inquiries from consumers, providers, and employers.
5. Provide on-line maintenance of files for members, consumers, providers, and physicians.
6. Obtain data for determining where to increase needed services.
7. Obtain wait time data to keep a finger on the pulse of access.

Source: Modified from documents produced at Group Health Cooperative of Puget Sound, Seattle, Washington.

Figure 16-3.   RMS Uses in Budget/Financial and Cost Management

1. Obtain data on incurred but not reported liabilities.

2. Provide early identification of potentially high-cost care.

3. Identify trends in high-cost services/excessive charges.

4. Provide variance data between actual billed charges and preauthorized estimates of charges by provider, patient, and services.

5. Provide data for contract negotiations and management for provider services.

6. Track "who's doing what on whose behalf" for budget planning and reconciliation.

7. Do validity checks on all claims against preauthorized referrals (patient, provider, service, diagnosis, date range).

Source: Modified from documents produced at Group Health Cooperative of Puget Sound, Seattle, Washington.

Like the simple presentation of other management control mechanisms, having an automated referral management system does not in and of itself produce the theoretical benefits. System functions and data bases need to be used thoughtfully by appropriate players within the organizations. Referral management systems do not resolve the conflicts often present, for example, between administrators and practitioners in the cost and quality management processes. Issues of practice style, ethics, and control will continue to be dealt with by people, not machines. How RMS and other cost and quality management tools are used in professional relationships to benefit consumers of health care is as much a determinant of system benefits as a system itself.

Relative to certain other health care information systems, referral management systems are not plentiful in the marketplace. Of those that do exist, design features do not reflect the test of time, and many are modified extensively to accommodate specific organizational circumstances. For the seeker of referral management systems, it is important to know that they are not always marketed or identified as such. Often, for example, referral management systems functionality is found as the service preauthorization component of more comprehensive claims processing or managed care systems. (For a report that compares various managed care systems and vendors in the marketplace, see Singer, C. J. *Managed Care: Information Systems Vendors.* Marblehead, MA.) Several sources for referral management and service preauthorization functionality are listed below:

CSC Comtec, 34505 West Twelve Mile Road, Suite 300, Farmington Hills, MI 48331, 313/553-0900

IDX, 1500 Shelbourne Road, P.O. Box 1070, Burlington, VT 05402-1070, 415/569-6120; 800/468-4411

Orbis Peabody Group, Inc., 20 Catamore Boulevard, East Providence, RI 02914, 401/431-0900; 800/423-7088

Q-Care, 4525 Vineland Road, Suite 202, Orlando, FL 32811, 800/777-0757

Seako Managed Health Care Systems, 517 Beacon Parkway West, Birmingham, AL 35209, 205/945-8200

Tingley Systems, Inc., Highway 52 West, P.O. Box 700, San Antonio, FL 33576, 904/588-2250

Chapter 17

Appointment Scheduling

Lisa Osteraas and Matthew Kelliher

The experience of Harvard Community Health Plan (HCHP), a not-for-profit health maintenance organization (HMO) headquartered in Boston, illustrates a step-by-step approach to implementing an automated appointment scheduling process. A list of appointment scheduling vendors appears in appendix B.

Background on Harvard Community Health Plan

Harvard Community Health Plan has approximately 380,000 enrolled members and is the largest of New England's HMOs. Harvard Community Health Plan is a combination staff model (Health Center Division) and group model (Medical Groups Division) HMO and currently operates 23 separate sites that employ over 4,000 full-time staff and provide approximately 2 million ambulatory care visits annually.

Harvard Community Health Plan offers comprehensive health care services to its members in return for a prepaid fixed fee, plus a copayment on a per-visit basis. Services are provided at HCHP health centers, medical groups, affiliated hospitals, and HCHP designated providers.

Each member is encouraged to select an ambulatory care delivery site as their primary locale for the receipt of services. Upon selection, the member is further encouraged to choose a physician as their responsible primary care provider.

Health centers have many different clinical departments (for example, internal medicine, pediatrics, OB/GYN, and so forth), which can consist of one or more clinical units. A clinical unit is usually represented by two groups of three to four providers who practice as a team. Assisting these teams are clinical practice assistants (CPAs), nonmedically trained support staff who assist clinicians in conducting examinations, escorting patients, handling telephone calls, and scheduling appointments. The general operations and support staff in each clinical unit are managed by the clinical supervisor. If a clinical department consists of more than one clinical unit, the entire clinical department is managed by a clinical manager.

Current Systems

The following sections will outline the appointment scheduling environment at HCHP. Within HCHP exist both manual and automated appointment scheduling systems, each with its own advantages and disadvantages.

Problems with Manual Scheduling

Harvard Community Health Plan schedules appointments manually in all but one of its health centers. Appointments cannot be scheduled until appointment pages are made up and put into the appointment books. This is usually done three to four months in advance. The clinicians must first turn in their leave requests to the clinical supervisor, who then puts together a schedule of availability, keeping in mind that the unit must be adequately covered at all times. The on-call schedule is then developed from this master schedule. The appointment pages are made up (one for each half-day) and entered into the appointment binders, with one binder for each clinician. This entire process, including numerous changes once the pages are in the book, is very labor-intensive and time-consuming for the supervisor, taking approximately three full days per month.

Once the appointment pages are in the books, the clinical practice assistants can book appointments. Appointments are normally booked either over the phone or in person by the member. In order to determine availability for a certain physician at a certain time, the CPA must manually flip through that physician's book. For certain appointment types, such as physicals, which are booked far in advance, the process of finding an open slot is like finding a needle in a haystack. A physician's appointment book can only be accessed by one CPA at a time, yet two CPAs normally schedule four to five physicians. This often causes delays in patient and process flow while a CPA waits for access to a book.

When an available appointment slot is finally found and agreed upon, the CPA must obtain the following information from the patient and write it onto the appointment page: the patient's name, medical record number, home and daytime telephone numbers, and a brief comment on the reason for the appointment. It is very difficult for the CPA to locate appointments unless the inquirer knows exactly when the appointment is and with which clinician.

Three days in advance, the appointment book pages for the day in question for each physician are removed from the appointment book and copied. One copy stays in the unit for scheduling appointments during the two days prior to the day in question. The original goes to the medical record department, where it is data-entered in the Automated Medical Record System (AMRS) so that it can be printed. During the two days prior to the scheduled day, any additions to the schedule are noted in red pen by the CPAs. These updated schedules are sent to the medical record department the day before; anything written in red pen is added to the schedule previously entered. Copies of the schedule are printed out the previous night, which also triggers printing of the medical record. The printed schedules and medical record are delivered to the unit early on the morning of the scheduled day; printed schedules are distributed to the clinicians, the receptionist, and the CPAs. Any same-day appointments are added to the CPA copy in pen, and the charts on those appointments are requested by filling out a request slip, which the medical record department picks up periodically. Some units have access to printers on which they can request charts to be printed right in the unit. It is very difficult for the clinicians and the receptionist to have a handle on the patient flow for the day because the schedule is constantly being updated without them being regularly notified.

As patients arrive, the receptionist marks them off on his or her copy and verifies their telephone numbers and addresses. Any updates to the patient's demographic information are written on a card by the receptionist or the patient and delivered to the main reception desk daily for input into the enrollment/billing system. If a patient cancels or does not keep an appointment, the CPA indicates this on the printed schedule. Any reports on cancellation rate, visit volumes, or any other reports the unit would like are usually done from these copies of the printed schedule, either by hand or on a spreadsheet.

To summarize, some of the main problems HCHP has experienced with scheduling appointments manually include the following:

- The process is time-consuming, labor-intensive, and repetitive.
- Access to the schedules is restricted to one CPA at a time.
- It is very difficult to do searches for appointment information with anything less than the date, time, and clinician for the specific appointment.
- Demographic information in the system cannot be updated immediately.
- Communication to unit staff of last-minute changes in the schedule creates significant amounts of work.
- Reports require much time, and the format of these reports can differ from unit to unit.

Problems with Automated Scheduling

One of the health centers, serving approximately 40,000 members, had an automated scheduling system already in place. A few years ago, HCHP installed an automated scheduling system to try to address some of the manual scheduling problems.

With the best intentions in mind, the project team interviewed many supervisors and managers to find out how appointments were currently being scheduled. An important consideration in the system being sought was that it run on the proper hardware that HCHP had in place. A system was selected that met all the requirements that had been set forth—it ran on the proper hardware, and it could support the way that appointments were currently being scheduled.

Unfortunately, what HCHP installed was an automated version of the way appointments had been scheduled before. The schedulers in the automated environment have just as many problems as the schedulers in the manual environment. Some of these issues include the following:

- When a study is completed in two different centers, it was found that it took just as long to schedule an appointment manually as it did using the automated system.
- The development of the providers' schedules is all done on paper until final approval, when the clinical supervisor in each department must enter the schedules into the system.
- Just as the manual schedulers have to flip through the entire book to find empty slots, the schedulers on the automated system have to flip through many different screens to ascertain the providers' availability.
- The system uses scrolling, and the scheduler has to type in a command to bring back any information that was previously on the screen.
- On the actual day of the schedule, any changes are made in pen on the printed copy. The receptionist marks off arrivals on the schedule using a pen, just as is done in the manual environment.
- Just as the manual schedulers have problems accessing the appointment books, the automated schedulers have access problems to the system's line into the mainframe.
- Many people have become more and more disillusioned with the efficiency of the automated system to the point where many of the physicians have begun to deinstall their schedules and go back to scheduling their appointments manually. Many of the clinical departments in the health center are maintaining two schedules, manual schedules as well as the automated schedules, effectively doubling the CPA's work load.

Between 1983 and 1987, HCHP membership grew rapidly. The organization was very busy trying to meet the demands of its continually growing membership and began to build many new health centers as quickly as possible. During this peak period, the Health Center Division became very concerned about the efficiency and overall quality of the service it delivered.

Model Clinical Unit Strategy

Health Center Division management commissioned the systems engineering department at HCHP to collaborate with management and staff at two representative clinical units to design a "model clinical unit." This model clinical unit design would be based on a profound understanding of the current primary care delivery system and include operational changes, facility designs, and recommendations for innovative support systems.

An internal medicine unit and a pediatrics unit at two separate health centers were selected to be analyzed. Video cameras were installed in the model units to assist in the initial process analysis. From these tapes, vital operational data such as waiting and service times as well as reason for visit and arrival distributions were gathered. Telephone call detail was captured, and systems engineering personnel spent considerable time at the two units doing extensive observations and interviewing staff throughout all levels of the two departments.

It was evident from the observations and interviews that the appointment and provider scheduling process was highly labor-intensive and time-consuming, whether manual or automated appointment scheduling was used in all of its ten health centers. The functional specifications for this system were developed based on this understanding of the current system and input from the people who actually schedule the appointments. Those same people were highly involved with the selection process from start to finish.

The automated scheduling system would be piloted in the two study units for an initial period to assess its impact and effectiveness and then, if the pilots were successful, the scheduling system would be gradually rolled out for use in all of the health centers.

When implementing a new appointment scheduling system, it is critical to have top-level commitment to the project from the start. Purchasing an automated appointment and provider scheduling system is a commitment that everyone in the company has made to improve clinical operations and service to its members. Because of this focus, the system must be owned not by management and not by data processing, but by the clinical departments themselves.

This process requires a great deal of time and effort from individuals at many different levels of the organization. It is very easy for the process to get bogged down in details and to get off on tangential tracks. That is why it is important that the first step that be taken once the working group is assembled is to develop a detailed project plan that outlines which tasks are to be performed, who the responsible party is, and what the expected dates of completion are. Appointing a user representative as project leader ensures that the needs of the users are always top priority. If the time is spent up front in agreeing to the plan and determining which individuals need to be involved, the project has a much greater chance for success.

To summarize, the major points of the new approach were:

- Major involvement from actual users
- Pilot of system before planwide implementation
- Top-level commitment
- Detailed planning from the start
- A user representative as project leader

Defining the Objectives

The first and most important step in the process was to define the needs of the users in detail. The group agreed that the basic objectives of purchasing a new system were user-oriented in nature and not management-oriented. The group felt that it was most important that the system make appointment scheduling easier and faster for the clinical practice assistants, the users who actually schedule the appointments all day every day. It decided that the principal focus should not be on data capture or what reports the system could provide for management.

The question at this point was: What information and tools do the schedulers need to schedule appointments quickly and easily? A logical way to start this process might be to go directly to the schedulers and ask them what they would change about it. Some good answers and ideas might come out of this, but it would be limited by the experience of the people who were asked. Instead of using this approach exclusively, HCHP developed functional requirements for its appointment scheduling system.

Functional Requirements for Appointment Scheduling

In order to prepare for the task at hand, the systems engineers involved had to become intimately familiar with the process of scheduling appointments. Many long hours were spent observing the schedulers and documenting the procedures they used. The engineers then drew up a preliminary list of what critical information the schedulers used and what additional information would be useful in scheduling. Then working meetings were held with clinical groups including supervisors, clinical practice assistants, and physicians to help detail the list. This list was thoroughly reviewed by staff at all levels in the health center, and additional information was added to form the functional requirements of the system. The functional requirements fell into seven major categories:

- *Provider scheduling.* This section included the requirements for scheduling which days and hours the providers would be available to see patients.
- *Appointment structure.* The appointment structure included the layout of the appointments. This was a critical section for HCHP because the providers did not just schedule appointments on fixed intervals, but used wave and pulse booking and combinations of the above.
- *Inquiry.* These requirements included which information was to appear when scheduling appointments and which information needed to be available but not necessarily displayed automatically.
- *Booking.* The booking section included the system requirements for the actual function of booking appointments.
- *Reporting.* Reporting, although not primary, was still an important requirement of the system.
- *Interfaces.* This section did not detail how the existing systems would interface with the automated scheduling system. This section merely outlined which information the automated scheduling system would need to get from other existing systems.
- *Backup and security.* How would the system provide backup and security?

Assessing the Marketplace

Parallel to this effort, a list of all vendors who offered automated scheduling systems was being researched (see appendix B). This list came from every source imaginable—from computer manufacturers' lists of software vendors to anything that was heard of by word of mouth. Because some of the people involved in the process had never been involved with automated appointment scheduling before, the systems engineering department and the clinical staff got together and attended a demonstration of one of the scheduling systems, selected randomly from the list that was being compiled. This helped tremendously to focus the effort and to lend hope that what was sought might actually be available.

Assembling the Task Group

When the functional specifications were still in the draft stages, a task group was formed to oversee the different efforts that were going on and to represent the different areas in making decisions on the direction and scope of the undertaking. The group included representatives from Health Center Division Operations, the medical systems management department (the department that would eventually maintain the software), and the systems engineering department, as well as a health center administrator. The group held regular meetings to process all the work that needed to be done and was responsible for including anyone throughout HCHP that the group felt should provide additional input.

Assembling the User Group

Because the group felt strongly that the focus needed to be on the user's needs, a user group was assembled to review the functional specifications and reporting requirements. The user group had representatives from all levels of the health center, including:

- Clinical practice assistants
- Physicians
- Clinical department supervisors
- Health center administrators

Not only was this group used to review and input, but also to keep the health centers involved in this acquisition and to keep everyone up to date on the process. When the functional specifications and the reporting requirements were finalized, then the user group was disbanded. Some members of the group became members in other smaller groups later on in the process.

The Request for Information

The next step in the process was to send a request for information (RFI) to the vendors that had been identified. Because the functional specifications had been finalized, it was important to find out how many vendors, if any, could provide the functionality that had been outlined and were interested in doing so. The preliminary list of 40 vendors had to be pared down to the key vendors who would receive a request for proposal (RFP).

The request for information should be a brief document that vendors can understand easily and respond to in an uncluttered, easily interpreted manner. The RFI, in this case, consisted of the list of the functional specifications with a request that the vendors specify which specifications their software could meet, which it could not meet, and which specifications their software could be modified to meet. The RFI also included a brief overview of HCHP and what was being sought and some short questions on hardware and system specifics. It was important to keep the RFI brief and to the point so that the group could garner the necessary information to make a preliminary decision without having to wade through 200 pages of information.

Once the responses to the RFI arrived, each member of the task group individually previewed the responses and assigned an overall rating to each system based on the functionality of the system. This was not an easy task. Some vendors had responded that they could meet every one of the 41 functional specifications that had been requested. What was the best way to judge a response such as this? Any system that got a highly unfavorable rating from all or most of the task group members was automatically eliminated from the process. The group was then assembled to discuss the remaining systems and to resolve any disparity in the ratings of those systems. Within the twelve finalists were systems that ran on many different machines. No system was rejected solely on the basis of incompatibility with current hardware and software. Simplifying the job of the schedulers was the first priority, and whichever system fit that objective best would be made to fit in with other HCHP systems.

The Vendor Review Team Approach

The task group was somewhat skeptical of certain vendor responses and also was aware of the complexity of the functional specifications and their susceptibility to misinterpretation. Therefore, the vendors had to be evaluated more closely. A vendor review team was assembled to conduct a systematic, hands-on assessment of the final twelve systems and narrow down the list to three to five vendors who would receive a detailed request for proposal. The vendor review team was a small core group of individuals that would remain consistent from demonstration to demonstration and would be able to dedicate a great deal of time to this task. The group had to be small so that they could discuss and evaluate, without too much difficulty and complexity, the demonstrations they attended.

The key components of this approach included:

- A small core group with technical and user representation to evaluate vendor demonstrations
- Much attention in the demonstrations to the functional specifications
- A strong desire to stick to the vendor review team agenda rather than to the vendor's agenda
- Extensive note taking during demonstrations

The final vendor review team had five members—a systems engineer, a clinical manager, two clinical practice assistants, and a technical representative from medical systems management. Before starting the demonstration review process, the group dedicated much time to familiarizing themselves with each and every functional specification. The review team also met and identified their goals and objectives in attending these demonstrations and committed to sticking to the team's agenda rather than letting the vendor set the pace.

One of the most important tools the vendor review team developed was a worksheet that organized the functional specifications and allowed team members to take notes during the course of the demonstration on the vendor's ability to meet each one. Every member of the review team was strongly encouraged to take notes on everything they saw and to ask questions of the vendor to clarify anything they saw.

The vendor review team met briefly after each demonstration to discuss among themselves what they had seen and to verbalize any general impressions. The team was able to agree verbally in some of these meetings on whether a system should receive further consideration. The team then had an extended session after all the demonstrations were complete to review all the demonstrations and decide which of the vendors would receive an RFP. Each functional specification was assigned a weight as to its importance in the overall success of the system. Each of the specifications was necessary, but some were more important than others. The team agreed on a rating for each system and its ability to meet each of the functional specifications. Ratings were multiplied by the specification's weight and were added together to form an overall score for the system. Amazingly enough, the three systems that became candidates to receive an RFP had very close scores; two were identical. The team then presented their method, final recommendations, and overall impressions to the task group.

The Request for Proposal Process

The key aspects of the request for proposal process were as follows:

- The RFP process was kept from top-level management.
- The RFP was approved by top-level management.
- The project team structure was reorganized.
- Followup demonstrations and site visits were held.

While the vendor review team was attending demonstrations of various scheduling software, the task group began assembling the RFP. The two processes were kept separate. In order to protect the review team from any bias and to give all vendors a fair chance, the task group did not hear anything about which vendors the review team liked until all of the demonstrations were complete. The RFP included many very detailed questions about the background and experience of the vendor, the system software, the application software, and the hardware and peripherals required. It also included the list of functional specifications once again and required detailed responses as to how the system met each one.

The RFP went through many revisions within the task group, and once the task group was satisfied with the content, the RFP was ready for internal review. It was reviewed by three vice-presidents and approved for distribution to the final three vendors. This was a major milestone in the project that everyone had worked very hard toward for the better part of a year.

Once the RFP had been sent out, it was time to look back on the accomplishments of the group thus far and to begin the even greater task ahead—selecting and implementing a system. At this stage in the process, the task group began to rethink its usefulness and effectiveness. As the work increased and the deadlines grew near, the task group had grown in size. It was becoming very difficult to schedule meetings and to come to decisions on issues. The group thought it was time to re-organize the structure of the task group and break it up into smaller, more focused groups.

Some of the members of the task group became members of a new project team. The project team added to its ranks a clinical manager and a clinical practice assistant. The project team would lead the effort during the selection and implementation phases. Members of the project team would lead groups of other HCHP individuals that would accomplish steps toward these goals. Examples of these smaller groups included a team to develop proposal evaluation criteria, a proposal review team, a team to develop recommendations for the training of users, and groups to lead technical and user implementation efforts. The other higher-level members of the task group formed a review board. They were director- and manager-level personnel and added to their ranks a health center administrator and a physician. The review team was responsible for reviewing the work put together by the project team and giving approval on decisions made by the project team such as the final vendor selected and the training plans for the users.

Followup Demonstrations and Site Visits

A selection team, led by members of the project team, was assembled to review the proposals in detail. This review process included visits to sites where each of the systems was installed so that the selection team could view the scheduling application of each system actually in use.

Prior to visiting these sites, the clinical practice assistants that were members of the selection team were assigned to come up with case studies or examples they found in their day-to-day scheduling of situations that came up often and were difficult to handle using current scheduling methods. The reference sites were presented with these case studies and asked to detail how the system in question would handle those situations.

Once the reference sites were visited and the selection team was comfortable with all aspects of the systems in question, the selection team presented these findings to the project team. The project team was responsible for studying the findings of the selection team and making a recommendation to the review board on which system should be selected. The review board's task was to understand and approve or reject the project team's recommendation. Once the review board approved the project team's recommendation, it was time to negotiate a contract with the vendor and begin detailed implementation planning.

Initial Planning for Implementation

Several issues must be addressed during preliminary planning for implementation of the new system. Detailed planning of system customization, implementation timetables, and user training should be done before pilot implementation is considered.

Once the decision to use a certain vendor was made, project team members contacted the selected vendor to begin detailed planning of system customization and the implementation timetables. This planning can be part of the contract process and should be begun immediately.

System Modification

System modification should be done in concert with the vendor to avoid the possibility of changing the software so that it is incompatible with future software releases. It is best for information systems purchases to minimize the amount of customization that they need to do on their own and do as much as possible with the vendor. The main reason for customization is to make the software compatible for interfacing with existing systems and to meet the needs laid out in the functional specifications.

User Training

The user training group should be assembled as soon as the RFP is issued. At HCHP, it included clinical practice assistants and clinical supervisors as well as representatives from corporate training and computer system training. This group should begin to develop user training outlines as soon as the RFP is sent out, and when selection of a vendor is made, the group should immediately begin to work with vendor training representatives to iron out details. The group's user training proposals at HCHP were subject to approval by the review board.

Pilot Implementation

Implementation of the new system was carried out in two major phases. The appointment scheduling system was first piloted in one to three representative sites for a specified time period. At the end of that time period, a decision was made that the pilot was successful, and then phase two began. This phase was a slow but steady rollout of the scheduling system to other areas of the delivery system.

Site Selection and Preparation

The system was to be piloted on a clinical unit level. This meant that two clinical departments in two different sites were selected to be the beta test sites. The pilots should be done at sites where the system has a reasonable chance of success, a site where the volume of appointments scheduled is high enough to challenge the system. The pilot should be uncomplicated. It should require few, if any, automated interfaces and minimal customization.

The pilot sites should be selected early on in the process so that staff in the pilot departments can be involved at every step—in developing the functional specifications, reviewing vendor demonstrations, and selecting the final system. This will reinforce that the system belongs to the clinical departments.

The pilot site staff should also be involved in planning the implementation and the training of the pilot site users. Proper training and practice time on the system is essential to its chances for success.

Evaluation of Success

Prior to installation in the pilot sites, the project team should begin to plan how to evaluate the success or the failure of the system in providing the benefits initially identified when the decision was made to automate appointment scheduling. This "acceptance test" should be part of the contract with the vendor. Once the automated appointment and provider scheduling system has been in place in the pilot sites for the previously determined time frame, the project team must make a recommendation to the review board as to whether the system should be rolled out to the rest of the plan or should be deinstalled. This recommendation is made as a result of data comparisons, as well as detailed input from pilot site staff.

Rollout

If the project team determines that the pilot has been a success and the review board agrees, the next step is to begin to systematically roll out the system to the rest of the sites. An example of how rollout might be accomplished follows:

A pilot site in this example is one of four internal medicine units in a health center. The next step would be to install automated scheduling in all of internal medicine at that center. Once the logistics of this move have been worked out, the next step would be to install the system throughout primary care (internal medicine and pediatrics) and then finally throughout the entire health center. At each step in the rollout process, there will be kinks that need to be worked out and procedural decisions that need to be made.

Once the system is up and running successfully in an entire health center, it is time to move on to the next health center. Implementation starts on the clinical level and works up through clinical department, primary care, and then the health center, as mentioned previously.

Conclusion

Harvard Community Health Plan concentrated on five major points in taking the above-described approach. Each point had a significant impact on the success of the acquisition and implementation of the automated appointment scheduling system. The five major points of this approach are:

- *Major involvement from actual users.* The focus of the entire process has been on the functionality of the appointment system and what major improvements that functionality can make to the appointment scheduling process in general. Having actual appointment schedulers closely tied to the process ensures that functionality remains a top priority.
- *Pilot of the system before organizationwide implementation of the system.* Piloting the system in isolated areas accomplishes two purposes. It ensures that the system meets all the criteria and is actually a feasible solution before the organization commits to a purchase for the entire delivery system. Piloting also provides the opportunity to work out any operational issues on a small scale with a minimal amount of upheaval to the rest of the organization.
- *Top-level commitment.* Top-level commitment, both to the approach the working group takes as well as to the decisions it makes, is essential to ensuring the working group's commitment to the project.
- *Detailed planning from the start.* A well-thought-out, detailed project plan is a fundamental part of any undertaking. With a project of this size and this importance, with working members of the team coming

from many different areas of the organization, a detailed project plan is a necessity.

- *A user representative as project leader.* The project leader's role is to coordinate each of these elements and ensure that they are included in each phase of the project. With a user representative fulfilling this role, the user's needs remain as the focal point of the process.

In acquiring an automated appointment scheduling system, there is always a chance that the system selected will be highly successful, no matter what approach is taken. By using this approach, however, HCHP believes that the chances of a successful implementation are that much greater.

Chapter 18

Outpatient Clinics

Ellen Marszalek-Gaucher

Ambulatory care is the major point of entry into the health care system and as such has great impact on the utilization of other health care services. It is helpful to conceptualize ambulatory care as a funnel controlling hospitalization (the most expensive health care resource), diagnostic and therapeutic procedures, rehabilitation, pharmaceuticals, and dental and visual services.

There is tremendous continuous pressure for change in the health care system, producing what is now a very dynamic environment of change in health care delivery. The health care consumers of today are sophisticated and have high expectations of health care providers. Today consumers demand a personalized approach, high-quality care, pleasant surroundings, and an affordable price from outpatient clinics. In order to compete effectively, most hospital-based ambulatory care departments have patterned themselves after the private practice model. In this model, each patient has an attending physician assigned to his or her care, and care delivered is comprehensive, with complete followup.

This chapter covers issues such as computer needs and wayfinding systems that are applicable to outpatient clinics. The experiences of the University of Michigan Hospitals will serve as one example of the kinds of information systems that can be implemented.

University of Michigan Hospitals Environment

The University of Michigan Hospitals (UMH) are constantly striving to improve services in order to compete effectively. Presently, UMH's ambulatory care services are housed in the A. Alfred Taubman Health Care Center, a $30 million building, which opened in February 1986 to demonstrate a commitment to high-quality practice in ambulatory care.

This building is designed with many patient amenities: an art program, both visual and performing arts, plants to soften the environment, elegant furnishings, a skylight for natural lighting, mirrored walls, and decentralized services to avoid queueing. The University of Michigan Hospitals have also expanded into satellite clinic systems to bring services closer to the customer. In essence, UMH is adapting to the changing delivery environment.

Computer Needs

Rapid expansion caused UMH to have many computer needs. It had to have a reliable means of setting up over 750,000 expected patient appointments with over 900 physicians, six days a week. Once a patient arrived, it needed a central registration function with the means to set up the patient record automatically and print face sheets and appointment slips. There also was a problem with using traditional signage programs to get patients and visitors through a complex geographic setting to their chosen destinations. A method was needed to interface with both the professional fee billing system and the hospital billing system. A system was needed that would track the medical record and facilitate its timely delivery to the site of patient care. Improved, faster communication tools were needed for patient care providers. A system was needed that would collect information in a manner that would enhance research, education, and management activities. All of these needs had to be integrated into a total system that provided high-quality care with a personalized, caring approach at a reasonable cost to the consumer and the institution in a convenient and readily accessible manner.

Through the coordinated efforts of Hospital Information Services, Ambulatory Care Services Administration, Inpatient Hospital Administration Services, and the leadership of the clinical departments of the University of Michigan Medical Centers, systems were designed to meet the needs of patients, administrative staff, and physicians.

Patient Management System

The platform upon which all of these systems are built is the Patient Management System. It is in this system that all the patient demographic information (name, age, address, date of birth, insurers, third-party payer, financial class), and any other particular, pertinent information about the patient is captured. By having this data in one data base shared by all other systems, it is possible to enjoy the economy of a single effort having multiple effects throughout other systems. In other words, any one person who has knowledge of new information about a patient can update that information in the Patient Management System, and all other systems are immediately notified of that change without the patient having to repeat any new information to each person they encounter throughout the patient care process.

Clinical Scheduling System

The Clinical Scheduling System is one of the systems that is based on the Patient Management System. The purpose of the Clinical Scheduling System is to facilitate the scheduling and maintenance of outpatient appointments at the University of Michigan Medical Center. The Clinical Scheduling System (CLS) maintains a computerized appointment book for each resource (which may be a physician, a room, or even a piece of equipment) that needs to have a separate schedule maintained for it. The appointment clerk has access to the patient data base for name, address, telephone number, birthdate, referring physician, and so forth. Before a new appointment is made, the CLS displays prior and existing appointments to prevent double-booking of a patient. The system facilitates the scheduling of multiple clinic visits on the same day and provides continuative care by identifying the resource that last attended the patient. It uses clinic wait lists to track requests for appointments when the exact resource, date, or time is not known; for example, for an annual visit. As the time for the appointment draws near, it reminds the clinics that these patients need appointments. The Clinical Scheduling System also allows for the grouping of resources and, during the appointment-making process, will search the appointment books of all the resources in a particular group, selecting the resource who is first available and least fully booked. Because the CLS has access to the patient data base, it also recognizes when reregistration is needed (currently every six months) and prints worklists so that registrars can preregister patients by telephone, thus saving patients time and effort when they come into the clinics. Other on-line functions allow for the revision of appointment data; the cancellation of appointments; the updating of appointment status to arrived, canceled, rescheduled, or no-show; and the printing of notices to be handed or mailed to the patient, which includes specific instructions, such as "Do not eat for 24 hours before your appointment" or "Please bring your medications with you." Appointments can be displayed by patient, by resource, and by clinic. Resource utilization, which is the comparison of booking limits versus the number booked, can be displayed month by month.

The Clinical Scheduling System provides functions to change the scheduling patterns of any resource, identifying appointments that need rescheduling because of pattern changes and entering them on a reschedule worklist. Appointments are rescheduled using on-line functions that copy all the appointment information to the new appointment time and mark the original appointment as having been rescheduled. The system generates automatic medical record pull slips, radiology film requests, and appointment reminder notices, relieving the appointment clerk from requesting these manually or via telephone. Other operational reports include the clinic and resource registers used to check patients into the clinic and alphabetical lists used by the information desks to direct patients to their appointments. The system provides managerial reporting that includes monthly resource utilization reports and monthly, quarterly, semiannual, and annual statistic reports. It is these data that allow administrators and clinicians to gather information to provide sound management judgments in the clinic or in inpatient areas and where more resources need to be devoted. These data allow researchers to identify particular types of patient populations in which they might have a particular study interest.

Wayfinding

Wayfinding has also been a huge problem for patient populations. The development and production of the wayfinding kiosk was carried out by a team composed of personnel from hospital information services, biomedical communications, and the medical wayfinding committee.

The purpose of the Wayfinder is to provide 24-hour-a-day assistance for visitors and patients to find locations in the University of Michigan Medical Center. The university medical center itself is quite large and is comprised of five major hospitals in separate buildings, a hotel, dozens of outpatient clinics, and clinical services, as well as shops and eating facilities. The location of the current Wayfinder, the first in a series planned for the medical center, is in the A. Alfred Taubman Outpatient Care Center at the University of Michigan Medical Center. The kiosk is located immediately to the right of the entry and exit point to the public parking structure. This is the major entry point of visitors and patients to the medical center complex.

The Wayfinder offers three services that are of value to hospital patients and visitors. It provides an audiovisual preview of the route and a hard-copy summary of route instructions, and it can also provide assistance in searching for the location of specific patients.

The most basic Wayfinder function is the route preview. The user selects his or her route via menus on a touch-screen. Once selected, the route is played back from video segments on the laser disk. Narration then points out landmarks, turning points, and the final destination. These video segments are interspersed with computer graphics, which display specific information, such as the correct floor on which to leave the elevator. When the audiovisual preview is finished, the user has three choices: repeat the preview, receive a hard-copy printout of route instructions, or simply leave the kiosk.

The second kiosk function is hard-copy printout. This contains a verbal description of the route. The kiosk user may request a printout at the end of the route preview. When the viewer has requested a destination for which a route preview is not available, a printout is automatically made. The hard-copy printout is produced on a laser printer driven by the Wayfinder computer, and the printout is ejected through a slot in the Wayfinder kiosk; a process that takes only a few seconds.

The last function of the Wayfinder is the Patient Locator. Here the user makes a choice, which turns the kiosk touch-screen into a keyboard facsimile. The user then enters the first and last name of the patient in question. If the patient is currently registered in the hospital, the screen displays the floor and area designation of the patient's room. The Wayfinder then asks if the visitor wishes instructions to that floor or area. Visitors are directed to the nursing center within the floor and area in order to protect patient privacy and promote a more orderly visitation policy.

Development and Evaluation

A limited program evaluation was conducted shortly after the wayfinding kiosk was installed. This survey found 94 users during a typical 24-hour period. Among surveyed users, 92 percent found the Wayfinder a significant help in finding their location. Seventy-nine percent of the users requested a printed copy of instructions in addition to the video. All of the users who found the Wayfinder of assistance said they would use it the next time they needed to find a location at the medical center.

On the basis of written evaluations that have been received, minor modifications are being made in the audiovisual routes of future wayfinding kiosks. Some users commented that they felt the routes were too long. An effort is being made to reduce the length of these routes. Long hallway shots are being shortened to reduce the timespan between important turning points and landmarks. These changes should increase the impact and memorability of the audiovisual segments.

Conclusion

The services provided by the patient management system, the clinical scheduling system, and the wayfinding kiosk have helped the University of Michigan Hospitals fulfill the high expectations of today's health care consumers. With these systems in place and with a continual evaluation of the changing marketplace, the University of Michigan Hospitals is effectively positioned for future outpatient clinic growth.

Chapter 19

Physician Office Systems

Elody F. Krieger

In today's world, physician practices are being forced to undergo computerization. Larger practices, larger patient data bases, more complex and varied insurance processing requirements, increased use of word processing, more complex appointment scheduling, electronic claims, and reimbursement freezes create a need for better and more efficient office procedures.

Computers can assist in office efficiency and enhanced profitability—both attractive to physicians and essential to their acceptance of computers. However, providing high-quality care for patients remains a physician's highest priority—and computers can assist with that too.

These needs create an opportunity for hospitals whose financial viability depends on a stable census. Hospitals can now enhance their relationship with community physicians by providing and marketing a variety of services to them. Computer systems technology currently offers one of the most promising means of meeting the physician's needs and the hospital's as well. This chapter describes the features, implementation challenges, and benefits of an automated communications link between physicians' offices and a hospital information system.

In an attempt to provide computer services to its medical staff, Children's Hospital, Columbus, Ohio, has developed a Physician Information Services Program to market and support computerized physician office systems and to provide the medical staff with a computerized link to Children's Hospital Information System (HIS). A coordinator was hired to write a business plan and implement the program.

Why the Program Was Needed

Children's became interested in this type of program for several reasons. First of all, it appeared that advances in the areas of telecommunications, microcomputer systems, and hospital information systems were providing Children's with the opportunity to improve pediatric patient care in central Ohio. Second, it was also clear that the expansion of the Children's Hospital Information System would make information available in an on-line mode—information that is critical to a physician's management of a patient's treatment. It was also known that Children's could easily and inexpensively link a computer system in a physician's office to the hospital mainframe. This type of access could result in tremendous improvement in the timeliness and accuracy of clinical information communications between physicians and the hospital. In addition, Children's realized that physicians lack both the time and expertise to search out computer system solutions for their practices.

The increasingly competitive health care environment was also factored into this decision. Although Children's is and was more immune to these pressures than most general care hospitals, it had a drop in average daily census of 12.9 percent between 1983 and 1985. As a result of even greater census declines, local general care hospitals had begun to retain and even recruit pediatric cases that they might previously have referred or transferred to Children's. Children's realized that it was important to strengthen its ties to the physician community in order to counteract this effect.

The provision of an automated communications link between a computer system in the physician's office and the HIS seemed an appropriately targeted program to accomplish this. Children's wanted to make it as convenient as possible for a physician to have a patient admitted to its hospital.

There was an additional incentive to move quickly with this program due to the interest of other hospitals in establishing a similar program. Although the concept of a hospital supporting a network of physician office systems was still fairly new, even at the national level, the interest was great enough that virtually every hospital in the Columbus area was evaluating such a move. Recognizing that the first hospital to succeed with this program would effectively "lock in" a portion of the marketplace, Children's decided to move as quickly as possible.

Hospitals and physicians both say that computer linkages are one of the most requested and unfulfilled services. But are hospitals planning to offer them? Recent studies indicate that more than one-fourth say "yea."

Children's Hospital Link

Children's chose to address both practice management computing and a link to the hospital system. This chapter will primarily address the Children's Hospital Link (CHL), which is now over two years old.

Although the CHL was designed solely for physician use and originally was geared to community-based physicians and their office personnel, Children's also had a large multispecialty medical practice located within the hospital that also expressed a strong interest in accessing the CHL. This internal group is now the primary user of the link service.

Physician Requirements

In the implementation of this program, Children's formed a physician office systems task force. This body included both administrators and medical staff members. The medical staff had two basic requirements in the development of a link. The first was that the link be available to any member of the medical staff regardless of the computer system used in their practice. The second requirement was that if Children's were to provide computer equipment to the physicians for remote access to Children's, that same equipment should be able to access other hospital links in the Columbus area as those links were made available.

In response to those requirements, Children's decided to make the link access as generic as possible. Terminal emulation provides inquiry capabilities for physicians and allows the vast majority of the dial-in users to access the link easily and inexpensively. The mainframe hardware includes MultiTech modems, an IBM protocol converter (7171), and a Digital Pathways call-back security system. The 7171 accepts a variety of common emulations.

Allowing any computer system to access its link limited Children's ability to perform uploading and downloading of information between the practice management system and the hospital system. Given that a large percentage of Children's admissions come from relatively few members of its medical staff, information passing was not perceived as a crucial element of its link service. As the link continues to grow, Children's hopes to offer information passing as an option to those practices that purchase their systems through the hospital.

Opening the CHL to all computerized practices also presented Children's with some advantages. Two other hospitals in the Columbus area also have physician practice management system programs. One has contacted Children's to determine the feasibility of allowing their physician offices to dial into the CHL. Thus, Children's "open access" policy allows other system vendors to use the CHL as a selling advantage to their systems.

Although this policy may reduce the number of practice management systems that Children's sells (systems sales are not-for-profit), it still accomplishes its goal of providing high-quality care (through easy data access) and strengthens its ties with the medical staff.

Even if another system vendor includes the CHL with their system, Children's is still responsible for training office staff on the use of the

CHL. By maintaining direct contact with the practice, Children's still benefits by providing the service.

Security

In addition to having open access to the CHL, physicians have unlimited access to patient data. Any physician with authorization to use the link can access any patient's information, regardless of the physician's activity with a particular patient. Limiting access to critical patient data was erceived by the physicians as a hindrance to high-quality patient care.

Rather than provide automatic access to all physicians, Children's requires physicians to request authorization to use the link. Forms are completed by a coordinator, and identification numbers and passwords are assigned by the information systems department for each physician and his or her staff. This process provides an opportunity for the coordinator to discuss the various options available to the practice for access to the CHL. These options include:

- Directing the physician to a local vendor to purchase recommended hardware (if computers are needed)
- Testing existing personal computer hardware for use with the link and recommending hardware options if existing equipment will not suffice
- Meeting with the practice's system vendor to discuss the requirements for access to the link

Finally, once the hardware has been tested and ID numbers and passwords are obtained, the practice is ready to "call" the CHL. In order to ensure that the caller is an authorized user, Children's uses a dial-back security device called the Defender, by Digital Pathways. This system requires the physician to call the computer system and enter a security code; both systems then "hang-up." About one minute later, Defender calls back to a predefined telephone number. Physicians can have access from their office or home; however, each location requires its own dial-back security code.

Features

When the link was first developed, the Hospital Information Systems (HIS) was a home-grown admissions/discharge/transfer (ADT) system; however, an HIS selection process was under way to replace that system. Because Children's anticipated that the then-current HIS hardware would not change dramatically with the software change, it decided to proceed with development of screen flows for the physicians.

Functions that are available via the original CHL included:

- Patient demographic and insurance information
- Patient case histories
- Patient rounds lists
- Patient insurance information
- Current inpatient listings
- Room/bed census by
  - Unit
  - Attending physician
  - Service area
  - Church code
- Preadmissions

In addition to basic ADT functions offered with the initial link, preadmissions was added specifically for physician use. Although this function is highly successful at other hospitals, it was not as successful for Children's. The reasons for its lackluster reception are probably twofold. The first is that those primarily accounting for the high rate of admissions at Children's are members of its internal group practice or they are surgeons. Both of these groups in most cases have already computerized (not with the system that Children's now recommends), and so uploading data (a prime advantage of computerized preadmission) from the physicians' computers is nearly impossible and has not been pursued to date.

Second, preadmissions is perceived to be more of a benefit to the hospital than to the physician's office staff. Thus, the physicians have not pursued access to the link due to the cost involved in purchasing modems and custom programming from their current vendors.

About six months after the initial CHL development, the Shared Medical Systems Independence software was chosen for Children's new HIS. Screen flows were rewritten for physician access on the system and were available when the system went "live" in November 1987. [In order to enter or retrieve specific information on a patient, you have to go through a certain number of screens (due to space limits for text per screen and a tiered structure), which can be very time-consuming.]

About three months after the implementation of the Independence system, Children's information systems staff were able to integrate the SMS software with the Community Health Computing laboratory system to make laboratory test results available over the link. Laboratory results generated a great deal of interest among the medical staff, and this has continued to be one of the more heavily utilized features of the link.

Another feature that was added later was electronic mail (EM). Although EM was perceived as a useful tool for physicians, Children's found that without a large core of internal physician users, the outside physicians had little incentive to use it. Since the implementation of EM, the number of internal physicians on the system has increased dramatically, and yet the number of external physicians who use it is still quite small. Plans are to continue the expansion of EM.

Desired Features

In a survey of physicians' interests in computerized links recently completed at Children's (table 19-1), the physicians indicated that their number one desire in the link was ancillary test status and results reporting. Their second most desired feature was access to patient histories. Although Children's had addressed both of these needs, there are a number of other areas that the hospital plans to address over the next two to three years.

The third most important function in a link, as expressed through the survey, was access to medical records transcribed reports. Children's is currently unable to offer these data on the CHL, but it is a function that will be investigated in the future.

Table 19-1. Physician Interest Survey

Using the scale below, please check your degree of interest in having any of the following computerized links to Children's Hospital from your office or home (response includes both computerized and noncomputerized practices).

	Very Interested (%)	Somewhat Interested (%)	Not Interested (%)	Interest Indicated (%)
Ancillary test status and results reporting	57.97	15.94	26.09	73.91
Patient history reporting	20.00	45.00	35.00	65.00
Clinic reports*	25.00	40.00	35.00	65.00
Consults*	25.00	40.00	35.00	65.00
Histories and physicals*	30.00	35.00	35.00	65.00
Discharge summaries*	30.00	35.00	35.00	65.00
Radiology reports*	30.00	35.00	35.00	65.00
Autopsy reports*	20.00	40.00	40.00	60.00
EEGs*	25.00	35.00	40.00	60.00
Electronic mail/consult requests	10.53	47.37	42.11	57.89
Patient demographics	21.05	36.84	42.11	57.89
Operative notes*	9.52	47.62	42.86	57.14
Order entry	10.53	42.11	47.37	52.63
Outpatient ancillary order entry	10.53	42.11	47.37	52.63
Emergency room preregistration entry	15.79	36.84	47.37	52.63
Preadmit patients via computer	5.26	42.11	52.63	47.37
Outpatient preregistration entry	10.53	36.84	52.63	47.37
Census data inquiry	11.11	22.22	66.67	33.33
Other	0.00	12.50	87.50	12.50

*Access to medical records transcribed reports.

Source: Children's Hospital, Columbus, Ohio, 1988.

Financing

The Children's Hospital Link is a free service that Children's provides to its medical staff. Once the physician acquires the computer hardware necessary to access the link, no further charges are incurred. Children's does not charge for time spent in making a physician's system operate properly with the link or for the physician's computer access time.

If a physician opts to purchase a practice management system from the hospital, the system price would typically include a modem to access the CHL. The system (hardware, software, modem, and so forth), which is sold at hospital cost, is then financed at prime plus one point over five years.

If the physician does not choose to purchase a practice management system, then he or she is asked to purchase the computer hardware. The hospital's personal computer vendor offers these systems at the same discount level achieved by the hospital. Financing options do not currently exist for these individuals; however, Children's is now reviewing this policy.

Children's has found that it needs to review its financing terms on at least a yearly basis to remain competitive in the marketplace. For example, at the time Children's implemented this program, its financing and purchase arrangements were quite competitive. However, these terms are now under review by Children's in light of better financing arrangements being offered by other area hospitals.

Challenges

The assistant executive director, information systems, cultivated and directed the development of the Physician Information Services program. As a result, the program was not only well received by administration (of which he is an active member), but was also well received by the data-processing department, which was heavily involved with the development of the CHL. This support was critical to the success of the program.

Even with that support, Children's recognized that there would be several challenges in integrating a physician's computer system with its Children's Hospital Link. They included:

- Obtaining administrative and medical staff approval
- Pricing the system
- Selecting and setting up hardware
- Customizing the system
  - Communications software
  - Physician screen flows
  - Ease of use

- Maintaining hardware/software link
  - Modems, protocol converter, and security device
- Training
- Marketing

Obtaining Approval

The first step in obtaining approval for the program was the development of a detailed business plan (figure 19-1). This plan included a description of the scope of the project, the benefits for the hospital and the physician, a market analysis, a description of the link, resources required, and a cost analysis.

This plan was presented to the information systems advisory committee. This committee is made up of senior administrative and medical

Figure 19-1. Business Plan

I. Executive overview

II. Background

III. Scope of project

    A. Local support efforts

    B. Hospital link

    C. Private practice computer system

IV. Program benefits

    A. The hospital

    B. The physician

    C. The computer vendor

V. Practice management system vendor

VI. Market analysis

VII. Support

VIII. Training

IX. Marketing

X. Children's hospital link

XI. System cost

XII. Resources required

XIII. System pricing

    Appendixes

    A—Training program

    B—Marketing schedule

    C—Physician survey results and analysis

    D—Vendor resume

    E—Sample license agreement

    F—Five-year financial worksheets for program

Source: Children's Hospital, Columbus, Ohio, 1988.

staff members who review the activities of the information systems area on a regular basis. After a review of the plan and an overview presentation of the material, the advisory committee recommended that the hospital proceed with the project, and the executive director approved the necessary funding.

Pricing the System

In developing the business plan, Children's needed to identify and project the cost of the program and evaluate financing alternatives. The recommendation that it felt would be most competitive and reasonable to the physicians was to sell the practice management system at cost without recouping its associated expenses. Because Children's had negotiated for substantial volume discounts for both hardware and software, this meant that the client practices would be able to acquire the system at a price far below retail.

To further enhance its objective to provide as attractive a package as possible for the physician, Children's also included a six-month, no-fault, money-back guarantee and an option to lease the system at a low financing rate.

However, these costs are associated more with the practice management system than with the CHL. As stated before, the link is a free service that Children's provides to its medical staff.

Hardware Selection and Setup

Once the program was approved, it was necessary to find and obtain hardware to facilitate the CHL. With virtually no telecommunications experts on staff, Children's had to rely on contacts in the community and on its vendor for recommendations. The practice management systems vendor was already experienced with the IBM 7171 protocol converter and with the Defender unit (a dial-back security device). This configuration was also recommended by other area corporations. Also recommended by vendors were 2400 baud error correcting MultiModems by MultiTech Systems.

The recommended hardware was purchased, and with assistance from the vendors, the hardware was operational in a short period of time. This configuration has proved to be fairly reliable.

Customizing the System

The system was adapted for CHL's needs by obtaining appropriate communications software, providing physicians with a unique set of menu screens, and making the dial-in process to the link easier to use.

Communications Software

In addition to hardware, communications software was necessary for the physicians to access the HIS. This software was either written or purchased for use on personal computers and on the practice management systems.

For users of personal computers with modems, Children's relied on the recommendations of its medical staff members and chose Mirror II communications software by Soft Klone. This package is regularly used by many of its medical staff members for on-line medical literature searches. Although several other communications packages are in use, Children's opted to support only one.

Many hospital personal computer users are also connected to the CHL via 3270 emulation/coax and via the hospital local network.

On the practice management system, the vendor was responsible for providing the practices with IBM 3101 emulation. This particular emulation was necessary because of its ability to perform the "cursor-select" function. Cursor-select is a key that emulates a light pen. Light pens are heavily used on the HIS.

Physician Screen Flows

In addition to communications software, a decision was made to provide the physicians with a unique set of screens on the HIS. These screens eliminated unwanted information and substantially increased the amount of physician/practice information. These screens also allow the physicians to review the information on any patient—screens for most other staff members are typically limited to the patients on a particular floor or unit.

Since the initial development of the link, many physicians who regularly use the CHL have provided Children's with invaluable feedback on their screens. As a result of their input, Children's has been able to streamline the screens to provide the same information in a more concise fashion. Requests for the expansion of link information are also regularly received.

Ease of Use

Making the system easy for the physicians and their staffs to use was a prime consideration in the development of the CHL. Providing physicians with unique screens in part addressed this goal.

However, the dial-in process itself was difficult. In order to reduce the chance of errors during the dial-in process, Children's developed customized script (batch) files for use with the Mirror II software. These files have the dial commands and remote access code necessary for accessing the link. These script files eliminated much of the frustration encountered in establishing the link manually.

Maintaining the Children's Hospital Link

Maintenance of the Children's Hospital Link involved developing modem standards and periodically checking the protocol converter and the dial-back security device.

Modems, Protocol Converter, and Security Device

As indicated previously, one of the most frustrating pieces of the link was establishing the modem connection. In order to reduce frustrations and the amount of time invested in testing modems and communications software, Children's developed modem standards. The modems that were tested and are currently supported included Hayes, MultiTech, and Everex.

These modems are now recommended to anyone who is considering use of the link. This is not to say that other modems will not work or that an attempt will not be made to interface other, nonstandard modems; however, it means that Children's will spend a minimum of time in testing them.

Some hospitals that are transferring data between systems (as opposed to inquiry-only systems) have resorted to leased telephone lines to manage their link. With Children's current volume and the relatively few practices that actually input data, leased lines are not yet justified.

Other than modem connections, neither the 7171 protocol converter nor the Defender unit has proved to be particularly difficult or time-consuming to maintain. Nor does either seem particularly prone to errors. Both pieces are effectively supported by the technical support staff or operations manager.

Training

Another responsibility in establishing a link is to provide training to physicians and their staff. Once again, the greatest difficulty comes in effectively training them in contending with modem problems. A large part of the training includes teaching the staff to recognize when dialing errors occur and giving them directions on clearing an error and restarting the dial-in process.

Training on the use of the HIS takes about one hour. A short manual accompanies the training. The manual includes dial-in, log on, log off, and laboratory inquiry directions. In addition, there are two definition manuals that elaborate on the definitions used throughout the system.

Marketing

Marketing has proved to be one of the most difficult tasks in establishing the CHL. This is in part because marketing is a rather new phenomenon for Children's and, given the multiplicity of projects on the marketing department's schedule, the CHL has received a rather low priority.

Another marketing factor is that because they are a prime target for marketing campaigns from so many different vendors, physicians, in order to defend themselves, have become a very difficult market to reach. Staff often provides a wall for defense that prevents marketing material ever reaching a physician's desk. In addition, most physicians have little time to spend in analyzing computer systems, so demonstrations must be quick and to the point—a difficult task for a complex technology.

Marketing campaigns directed to the office staff have proved to be effective, but it is the physician who typically makes the purchase decisions for the practice. Thus, even though an interest may be sparked in the office staff, marketers must still gain the attention and interest of the physician.

Although Children's practice management system vendor provides a marketing representative to market its system (which includes the link), the vendor often relies on the hospital to develop the market and provide the prospects. In addition, this representative is not responsible for sales that involve the link alone. The marketing strategies employed by the representative often mirror those being successfully used at other hospitals—they have not proved to be as effective at Children's.

Some of the marketing techniques employed have included:

- CHL/practice management system seminar
- CHL/practice management system breakfast meeting
- Medical section meeting presentations
- Attendance at monthly medical department staff meetings
- Attendance at quarterly general medical staff meetings
- Monthly CHL demonstrations in physician lounge
- Advertisements in Academy of Medicine Directory
- Direct mail
- Attendance at monthly pediatric office manager's meetings

Because these marketing techniques have been primarily responsible for most of the CHL installations and the practice management system sales, they could be considered successful. However, sales and installations are lower than originally anticipated.

CHL Advantages

The advantages in a link service are different for the hospital and for the physician.

Advantages for the Hospital

The advantages for the hospital include marketing edge, increased admissions and improved physician loyalty, improved patient care, and improved communications.

Marketing Edge

By offering the link in the Columbus market, Children's has a marketing edge over the general care hospitals. General care hospitals are usually interested in bonding the physician to only their hospital and typically will not allow systems supplied or purchased through them to link to any other general care hospital. Because Children's is willing to extend its systems to utilize any hospital's link, a physician should be more likely to choose Children's link before another hospital's more limited one.

In addition, the general care hospitals are likely to include a link to Children's with the system they market, because virtually all of these hospitals have pediatricians on staff who would find that access necessary. This gives CHL access to any physician who desires it.

Increased Admissions and Improved Physician Loyalty

A marketing advantage often realized by general care hospitals is an increase in admissions. It is said that "one extra bed filled per day for a year in the hospital could recoup more than the investment of time and resources for an entire (computer) system." Although increased or stable admissions is a potential benefit to Children's, it is not one of the primary goals at Children's, nor is the CHL expected to have a great deal of impact on admissions. The CHL should help to bond the physician to Children's and create a greater physician dependency on the hospital and the service it provides.

Improved Patient Care

Children's patients should be the primary benefactor of the CHL. If a physician is able to quickly access and review information particular to the patient and the patient's case, then the physician will be able to provide a higher level of care for the patient.

Improved Communications

The CHL has already proved to be effective in improving the flow of information between the hospital and the physician. Physicians and their staffs who use the link are already finding the easy access of information to be invaluable in their workday. Terminals located in the physician lounge, in their offices, and on the patient floors are being used primarily to access laboratory results, room and bed information, preadmissions, and billing data. All of this information could be transmitted by using the telephone, but this group chooses to use the CHL.

Advantages for the Physician

Vendors are constantly pursuing physicians to buy a computer system. Computers are a major investment for any physician. Legitimately, some physicians now ask, "What is the computer going to do for me?" or "How is this computer going to improve the care I can provide to my patients?"

The CHL is a direct benefit to the physician. For example, one problem identified by physicians is that on occasion a patient is discharged and yet still has outstanding laboratory tests. When the tests are complete, the result is placed in the chart. Unless the physician remembers that the tests are outstanding and remembers to order the chart, the test result is not reviewed. With the CHL, the physician can see all patients discharged over a specified period of time and request laboratory results that were posted after the discharge date.

Another benefit of on-line laboratory tests is that just prior to a patient's followup visit following discharge, test results pertinent to the visit can be reviewed and printed as a permanent addition to the patient's chart.

Conclusion

Although the Children's Hospital Link has been successful, the emphasis of its program to date has been on practice management systems. The link has been secondary. Children's continues to maintain its commitment to practice management systems, but it is currently placing more time and effort in marketing and supporting the link on a standalone basis.

Children's believes that the Children's Hospital Link provides it with the opportunity not only to serve its most important resource—its physicians—but also to continue in its endeavor to provide excellence in patient care.

Appendix A

Ambulatory Care
Vendor Listing

The *Ambulatory Care Vendor Listing* was prepared by Sheldon I. Dorenfest & Associates, Ltd. This listing is intended to be for information use only. It is not meant to be a complete listing of computer software vendors, nor does it imply the endorsement or recommendation of the listed companies by Sheldon I. Dorenfest & Associates, Ltd., or the American Hospital Association.

This listing was prepared using three main sources of information:

- *Computer Vendors for Group Practice,* developed by the Library Resource Center of the Medical Group Management Association, June 1988 edition.
- *Computers in Healthcare, 1988 and 1990 Market Directories,* Cardiff Publishing Company.
- Research performed by Sheldon I. Dorenfest & Associates, Ltd., for development of a presentation on the review of the ambulatory care information systems marketplace. This presentation was made in a seminar sponsored by the Healthcare Information and Management Systems Society and the Society for Ambulatory Care Professionals of the American Hospital Association.

Estimates show that there are well over 1,000 vendors servicing various areas and applications of the ambulatory care and group practice systems marketplace. This listing includes approximately 140 of these vendors, who were chosen based on their apparent breadth of functionality, services offered nationwide, and group size range.

In the vendor profiles an attempt has been made to offer insight into the applications and functionality each vendor provides. Depending on the source of information, the level of detail will be different. A vendor profile with a brief application list may in fact offer a wide and full range of functionality.

The following list depicts some of the key functions/applications offered in today's systems:

- Accounts receivable (AR)
- Appointment scheduling
- Billing (point of service, cycle, and so forth)
- Registration
- Accessible patient demographics/history
- Automated medical records/chart tracking
- Patient recall
- Collections
- Electronic claims
- Hospital–physician link
- Financial and clinical integration
- Management reporting
- General accounting (general ledger, accounts payable, fixed assets)
- Prepaid/HMO/PPO/IPA reporting
- Forecasting/financial modeling
- Inventory/purchasing

The *Ambulatory Care Vendor Listing* will aid in the search for a new software vendor. Readers are advised to contact these firms on an ongoing basis because relevant source information may be revised frequently.

Advanced Institutional Management Software, Inc. (AIMS)

Address:	485 Underhill Boulevard, Syosset, NY 11791-3414
Phone:	516/496-7700
Hardware:	IBM System 36, AS/400, PC, XT, AT, PS2
Group Size Range:	Not available
Suggested Group Size:	Not available
Applications:	Physicians' office management, scheduling, and billing

AISCorp

Address:	225 Jackson Street, Bridgewater, NJ 08807
Phone:	800/AIS-CORP; 201/526-8100
Hardware:	DEC PDP II and VAX
Group Size Range:	Unlimited—largest system currently installed handles 350 physicians
Suggested Group Size:	350 physicians
Applications:	Accounts payable, appointment scheduling/recall, billing/AR, collections, demographics,

electronic claims, general ledger, hospital–
physician link, hospital tracking, inventory/
purchasing, management reporting, medical
records, multiple payer privileges, patient
registration and history, payroll, personnel
management, physician productivity,
spreadsheets, word processing

Allen Associates, Inc.

Address: 968 Main Street, Box 3122, Wakefield, MA
                      01880
Phone: 617/245-5974
Hardware: DEC, IMP PC, XT, AT
Group Size Range: Small to large
Suggested Group Size: Not available
Applications: Physician office management, billing,
                      appointment scheduling, clinical and other
                      applications such as mental health and
                      home health care systems

American Business Computers, Inc.

Address: 140 North Highway 227, P.O. Box 936,
                      Clute, TX 77531
Phone: 409/265-2573; 800/237-5036
Hardware: DEC and IBM PC compatibles
Group Size Range: 1 to large
Suggested Group Size: Not available
Applications: Physician office management, billing, clini-
                      cal appointment scheduling, hospital–physi-
                      cian link

American Digital Systems Corporation

Address: 8401 Arlington Boulevard, Fairfax, VA 22031
Phone: 703/876-4760
Hardware: Altos, IBM PC, AT
Group Size Range: Any size
Suggested Group Size: Any size
Applications: Physician office management, billing,
                      appointment scheduling, clinical systems

American Medical Software, Inc.

Address: 5450 Peachtree Parkway, Suite 2A59,
                      Norcross, GA 30092
Phone: 404/448-6613
Hardware: Not available
Group Size Range: Small to large

Suggested Group Size: Small to large
Applications: Physician office management, AR, billing
                        options, electronic claims, appointment
                        scheduling, clinical and other applications

American Physicians Service Group, Inc.

Address: 1301 Capitol of Texas Highway, Suite B220,
                        Austin, TX 78746
Phone: 512/328-0888; 800/252-3628
Hardware: HP 3000
Group Size Range: 20 to 1,000
Suggested Group Size: More than 20 physicians
Applications: Accounts payable, appointment scheduling/
                        recall, billing/AR, chart tracking, collections,
                        demographics, electronic claims, fixed assets,
                        forecasting/modeling, general ledger, hospital–
                        physician link, hospital tracking, income
                        distribution, inventory/purchasing, manage-
                        ment reporting, medical records, multiple
                        payer privileges, patient registration and
                        history, payroll, personnel management,
                        physician productivity, prepaid/HMO
                        reporting, prescription tracking, spread-
                        sheets, utilization review, word processing

Andent, Inc.

Address: 1000 North Avenue, Waukegan, IL 60085
Phone: 708/223-5077
Hardware: Not available
Group Size Range: Solo – small
Suggested Group Size: Not available
Applications: 28 application modules for physician office
                        management, including appointment sched-
                        uling, billing, and clinical and billing
                        applications

APS/Databill, Inc.

Address: 21201 Oxnard Street, Woodland Hills, CA
                        91367
Phone: 818/716-9600
Hardware: IBM, NCR, Honeywell-Bull, HP
Group Size Range: 1 to 100-plus
Suggested Group Size: 1 to 20 physicians
Applications: Accounts payable, appointment scheduling/
                        recall, billing/AR, collections, demographics,

electronic claims, fixed assets, general ledger, hospital–physician link, income distribution, inventory/purchasing, management reporting, medical records, multiple payer privileges, patient registration and history, payroll, physician productivity, prepaid/HMO reporting, prescription tracking, spreadsheets, utilization review, word processing

APS Systems

Address:	4240 Piedras Drive, Suite 200, San Antonio, TX 78228
Phone:	512/736-2871
Hardware:	IBM and compatibles, NCR, TI, Compaq
Group Size Range:	Not available
Suggested Group Size:	1 to 99 physicians
Applications:	Accounts payable, appointment scheduling/recall, billing/AR, chart tracking, collections, demographics, fixed assets, general ledger, hospital tracking, income distribution, inventory/purchasing, management reporting, patient registration and history, payroll, personnel management, spreadsheets, utilization review, word processing

AR/Mediquest, Inc.

Address:	6105 West St. Joseph, Lansing, MI 48917
Phone:	517/323-0900
Hardware:	IBM System 36
Group Size Range:	Not available
Suggested Group Size:	Not available
Applications:	Physician office management, billing, clinical, appointment scheduling, physician link, and other applications

Articulate Publications (A Division of CyCare Systems, Inc.)

Address:	21201 Oxnard Street, Woodland Hills, CA 91367
Phone:	213/871-1350; 800/456-0708
Hardware:	IBM PC compatible – NOVELL Networking
Group Size Range:	Small to large clinics and physician office
Suggested Group Size:	Not available
Applications:	Physician office management, billing, appointment scheduling, physician–hospital link

Artificial Intelligence, Inc.
Address:	P.O. Box 569, Renton, WA 98057
Phone:	206/271-8633; 206/228-4667
Group Size Range:	1 to 99
Suggested Group Size:	5 to 10 physicians or dentists
Applications:	Billing/AR, collections, demographics, management reporting, multiple payer privileges, patient registration and history, physician productivity, prepaid/HMO reporting, word processing

AT&T
Address:	100 Southgate Parkway, Morristown, NJ 07960
Phone:	201/898-8176
Hardware:	AT&T 3B2 family
Group Size Range:	Not available
Suggested Group Size:	Not available
Applications:	Physician office management, billing, clinical appointment scheduling

Automated Medical Systems, Inc.
Address:	841 Chestnut Street, Suite 1310, Philadelphia, PA 19107
Phone:	215/923-1010
Hardware:	IBM, AT&T, Unisys, Rexon, Concurrent
Group Size Range:	1 to 200-plus
Suggested Group Size:	Hardware dependent
Applications:	Accounts payable, appointment scheduling/recall, billing/AR, chart tracking, clinical applications, collections, demographics, electronic claims, general ledger, hospital–physician link, hospital tracking, income distribution, management reporting, medical records, multiple payer privileges, patient registration and history, payroll, physician productivity, prepaid/HMO reporting, prescription tracking, spreadsheets, utilization review, word processing

Baxter Healthcare Corporation, Annson Systems Division
Address:	707 Skokie Boulevard, Suite 700, Northbrook, IL 60062
Phone:	708/564-8310
Hardware:	IBM PC, PS2, and System 36

Group Size Range:	1 to 25 (2 software packages, one for smaller and one for larger practices)
Suggested Group Size:	1 to 25 physicians
Applications:	Accounts payable, appointment scheduling/ recall, billing/AR, chart tracking, clinical applications, collections, demographics, electronic claims, general ledger, hospital–physician link, management reporting, medical records, multiple payer privileges, patient registration and history, payroll, personnel management, physician productivity, prepaid/HMO reporting, spreadsheets, utilization review, word processing

Biovation, Inc.

Address:	875 Alfred Nobel Drive, Hercules, CA 94547
Phone:	415/724-7290
Hardware:	Altos and AST PC
Group Size Range:	4 to 150
Suggested Group Size:	6 to 150 physicians
Applications:	Clinical applications

Business Computer Applications, Inc.

Address:	5515 Spalding Drive, Suite 109, Norcross, GA 30092
Phone:	404/263-6499
Hardware:	IBM System 3X
Group Size Range:	Small to large clinic
Suggested Group Size:	Not available
Applications:	Outpatient administration system including physician billing, appointment scheduling, and clinical applications

Calyx Corporation

Address:	150 North Sunnyslope Road, Brookfield, WI 53005
Phone:	414/782-0300
Hardware:	Altos, DEC, Wang, Compaq, HP, IBM, NEC, AT&T
Group Size Range:	Limited only by hardware on which it's running
Suggested Group Size:	Depends mainly on the hardware selected
Applications:	Accounts payable, appointment scheduling/ recall, billing/AR, collections, demographics,

electronic claims, general ledger, management reporting, medical records, multiple
payer privileges, patient registration and
history, payroll, physician productivity,
prepaid/HMO reporting, word processing

Care Information Systems, Inc.
Address:	P.O. Box 11140, Springfield, IL 62791
Phone:	217/529-0255
Hardware:	DEC PDP and VAX
Group Size Range:	Small to large
Suggested Group Size:	Not available
Applications:	Physician office management, billing, appointment scheduling, and physician–hospital link and clinical applications

C. M. Computers, Inc.
Address:	15220 32nd Avenue, South, Suite B, Seattle, WA 98188
Phone:	206/241-1199
Hardware:	IBM and CMC's own compatible
Group Size Range:	Up to 44 users
Suggested Group Size:	Any that require 44 or fewer serial ports
Applications:	Accounts payable, appointment scheduling/recall, billing/AR, chart tracking, clinical applications, collections, demographics, electronic claims, general ledger, hospital tracking, inventory/purchasing, management reporting, medical records, multiple payer privileges, patient registration and history, payroll, physician productivity, prepaid/HMO reporting, spreadsheets, utilization review, word processing

Collaborative Medical Systems
Address:	246 Walnut Street, Newton, MA 02160
Phone:	617/964-7880
Hardware:	DEC PDP 11 and VAX series, HP, Unisys, 286 and 386 PCs
Group Size Range:	Unlimited
Suggested Group Size:	Unlimited
Applications:	Accounts payable, appointment scheduling/recall, billing/AR, collections, demographics, electronic claims, general ledger, hospital tracking, income distribution, inventory/

purchasing, management reporting, medical records, multiple payer privileges, patient registration and history, payroll, personnel management, physician productivity, prepaid/HMO reporting, utilization review, word processing

Commercial Data Corporation, Health Care Systems Division

Address:	1177 Poplar Avenue, Memphis, TN 38105
Phone:	901/278-5800; 607/737-0458
Hardware:	Tandem, micros, and minis
Group Size Range:	Any size
Suggested Group Size:	Not available
Applications:	Physician billing

Computer Services Corporation

Address:	P.O. Box 10447-A, Midtown Center, Birmingham, AL 35202
Phone:	800/525-3635
Hardware:	IBM 4381, System 38 or PC, AT, RT
Group Size Range:	Not available
Suggested Group Size:	Not available
Applications:	Physician office AR, billing, and clinical applications

Computing Services, Inc.

Address:	8275 Melrose, Lenexa, KS 66214
Phone:	913/888-1050
Hardware:	Data General MV Series and desktops
Group Size Range:	Not available
Suggested Group Size:	Not available
Applications:	Patient, clinical, AR, insurance management, N.E.I.C. claims, word processing, and spreadsheets

Consolidated Data Services

Address:	3110 Craig Road, Eau Claire, WI 54701
Phone:	715/832-6320
Hardware:	IWS, AWS, NGEN, SRP
Group Size Range:	Not available
Suggested Group Size:	Not available
Applications:	Physician office billing, scheduling, clinical, management reporting, collection letters, mailing labels, third-party claim forms

Coopervision Information Systems
Address: Green & Lincoln Street, Lansdale, PA 19446
Phone: 215/368-9650
Hardware: IBM PC, Data General, DEC
Group Size Range: 50 physicians
Suggested Group Size: 2 to 12 physicians
Applications: Accounts payable, appointment scheduling/
                                recall, billing/AR, chart tracking, clinical
                                applications, collections, demographics,
                                electronic claims, fixed assets, forecasting/
                                modeling, general ledger, hospital–physician
                                link, income distribution, inventory/pur-
                                chasing, management reporting, medical
                                records, multiple payer privileges, patient
                                registration and history, payroll, physician
                                productivity, prepaid/HMO reporting,
                                prescription tracking, spreadsheets, word
                                processing

C&S Research Corporation
Address: 210 Goddard Boulevard, King of Prussia,
                                PA 19406
Phone: 215/265-9118
Hardware: IBM, WYSE, Sperry, MAI Basic Four, NCR
Group Size Range: 1 to 200-plus
Suggested Group Size: 1 to 200-plus physicians
Applications: Accounts payable, appointment scheduling/
                                recall, billing/AR, chart tracking, clinical
                                applications, collections, demographics,
                                electronic claims, fixed assets, forecasting/
                                modeling, general ledger, hospital–physician
                                link, hospital tracking, income distribution,
                                inventory/purchasing, management report-
                                ing, medical records, multiple payer
                                privileges, patient registration and history,
                                payroll, personnel management, physician
                                productivity, prepaid/HMO reporting, pre-
                                scription tracking, spreadsheets, utilization
                                review, word processing

CSC Comtec
Address: 34505 West Twelve Mile Road, Suite 300,
                                Farmington Hills, MI 48331

Phone: 313/553-0900
Hardware: Honeywell Ultimate, DEC Ultimate (Pick
                     operating system), IBM Pick/370, Prime
                     Information
Group Size Range: 500
Suggested Group Size: 15 physicians
Applications: Accounts payable, appointment scheduling/
                     recall, billing/AR, chart tracking, clinical
                     applications, collections, demographics,
                     electronic claims, fixed assets, general
                     ledger, hospital tracking, income distribu-
                     tion, inventory/purchasing, management
                     reporting, multiple payer privileges, patient
                     registration and history, payroll, physician
                     productivity, prepaid/HMO reporting, spread-
                     sheets, utilization review, word processing

CyCare Systems, Inc.

Address: 4343 East Camelback Road, Phoenix, AZ
                     85018
Phone: 602/952-5300
Hardware: Honeywell, IBM, Wang
Group Size Range: Offer products to address the needs of the
                     1- to 5-physician group, the 5- to
                     20-physician group, the 20- to 100-physician
                     group, and the 100-plus group
Suggested Group Size: Separate systems with unique characteris-
                     tics for groups of various sizes
Applications: Accounts payable, appointment scheduling/
                     recall, billing/AR, chart tracking, clinical
                     applications, collections, demographics,
                     electronic claims, fixed assets, forecasting/
                     modeling, general ledger, hospital–physician
                     link, hospital tracking, inventory/purchasing,
                     management reporting, medical records,
                     multiple payer privileges, patient registra-
                     tion and history, payroll, personnel man-
                     agement, physician productivity, prepaid/
                     HMO reporting, utilization review

Database, Inc.

Address: 1803A Chapel Hill Road, Durham, NC
                     27707
Phone: 919/493-6969
Hardware: Any DEC VAX series

Group Size Range:	Unlimited
Suggested Group Size:	Unlimited—hardware tailored to any size group
Applications:	Accounts payable, appointment scheduling/recall, billing/AR, chart tracking, clinical applications, collections, demographics, electronic claims, fixed assets, general ledger, hospital–physician link, hospital tracking, management reporting, medical records, multiple payer privileges, patient registration and history, payroll, physician productivity, prepaid/HMO reporting, prescription tracking, spreadsheets, utilization review, word processing

Datamerica Corporation

Address:	7½ East Wall Street, Fort Scott, KS 66701
Phone:	316/223-0770
Hardware:	None; however, systems are limited to NCR Corporation hardware
Group Size Range:	Up to 100
Suggested Group Size:	15 to 35 physicians
Applications:	Accounts payable, appointment scheduling/recall, billing/AR, clinical applications, collections, demographics, electronic claims, fixed assets, general ledger, hospital–physician link, management reporting, multiple payer privileges, patient registration and history, payroll, personnel management, physician productivity, prepaid/HMO reporting

Data Solutions, Inc.

Address:	28949 Euclid Avenue, Wickliffe, OH 44092-2548
Phone:	216/944-7944
Hardware:	IBM PC, AT, XT
Group Size Range:	Not available
Suggested Group Size:	Not available
Applications:	Physician office management, billing, appointment scheduling, laboratory, and home health care applications

Data Strategies, Inc.

Address:	17150 Via Del Campo, Suite 203, San Diego, CA 92127

Phone: 619/451-0480
Hardware: IBM, AST, Compaq
Group Size Range: 200
Suggested Group Size: 1 to 200 physicians
Applications: Accounts payable, appointment scheduling/ recall, billing/AR, collections, demographics, electronic claims, fixed assets, general ledger, income distribution, inventory/purchasing, management reporting, medical records, multiple payer privileges, patient registration and history, physician productivity, word processing

Delta Computer Systems, Inc.

Address: P.O. Box 1824, Altoona, PA 16603
Phone: 814/944-1651; 800-444-1651
Hardware: IBM, Contel
Group Size Range: Physician office or clinics
Suggested Group Size: Not available
Applications: Turnkey physician office management supporting EXECU-FLOW software

DISC Computer Systems

Address: 3055 Old Highway 8, Minneapolis, MN 55418
Phone: 800/331-4479
Hardware: NCR
Group Size Range: 1 to 50
Suggested Group Size: 4 to 20 physicians
Applications: Capitation, Report Writer, accounts payable, appointment scheduling, recall, billing, AR, chart tracking, collections, demographics, general ledger, income distribution, insurance claims, management reporting, patient registration, payroll, word processing

Dynamic Applications, Inc.

Address: 157 Engle Street, Englewood, NJ 07631
Phone: 201/569-2558; 800/633-4777
Hardware: Prime
Group Size Range: Physicians' offices and clinics
Suggested Group Size: Not available
Applications: Physician office management, billing, and appointment scheduling

EDP Systems, Inc.

Address:	720 East Park Boulevard, Suite 202, Plano, TX 75074
Phone:	214/881-8454
Hardware:	DEC VAX, IBM System 36
Group Size Range:	Limited only by size of hardware configuration; 50-plus physicians
Suggested Group Size:	Limited by hardware
Applications:	Accounts payable, appointment scheduling/recall, billing/AR, chart tracking, collections, demographics, electronic claims, forecasting/modeling, general ledger, income distribution, inventory/purchasing, management reporting, medical records, multiple payer privileges, patient registration and history, payroll, physician productivity

Elcomp Systems

Address:	Foster Plaza VI, 681 Anderson Drive, Pittsburgh, PA 15220
Phone:	412/937-0690; 800/441-8386
Hardware:	Data General minis, micros, and IBM PCs
Group Size Range:	Small to large
Suggested Group Size:	Not available
Applications:	Appointment scheduling, referral tracking, HMO/PPO Reporting, hospital tracking, inventory control, encounter forms, billing, AR, patient recall, insurance claim designer, word processing, payables, general ledger, payroll, electronic claims, marketing module, and management reporting

Encore Associates, Inc.

Address:	4354 South Sherwood, Suite 125, Baton Rouge, LA 70816
Phone:	214/243-7591; 504/291-7080
Hardware:	IBM System 36
Group Size Range:	2 to 60 physicians
Suggested Group Size:	3 to 40 physicians
Applications:	Accounts payable, appointment scheduling/recall, billing/AR, chart tracking, collections, demographics, electronic claims, general ledger, hospital–physician link, hospital tracking, income distribution, inventory/

purchasing, management reporting, medical records, multiple payer privileges, patient registration and history, payroll, personnel management, physician productivity, prepaid/HMO reporting, spreadsheets, utilization review, word processing

Enter Corp
Address:	2600 North Loop West, Suite 240, Houston, TX 77092
Phone:	713/683-2100; 800/231-0709
Hardware:	WYSE PC 286
Group Size Range:	Solo to multiuser small group practice
Suggested Group Size:	Not available
Applications:	Physician office management, billing, AR, and appointment scheduling

Epic Systems Corporation
Address:	5609 Medical Circle, Madison, WI 53719
Phone:	608/271-9000
Hardware:	Not available
Group Size Range:	Solo through large group practice
Suggested Group Size:	Not available
Applications:	Physician office management system, billing, AR, clinical, and appointment scheduling

Far West Systems
Address:	21201 Oxnard, Woodland Hills, CA 91367
Phone:	818/703-1186
Hardware:	Not available
Group Size Range:	Not available
Suggested Group Size:	Not available
Applications:	Practice management system including billing, AR, clinical, appointment scheduling, insurance tracking and posting, electronic claims

Fiscal Information, Inc.
Address:	985 Wilson Avenue, Loveland, CO 80537
Phone:	303/669-4340; 800/525-5370
Hardware:	Point 4 Data Corporation multiuser, multitasking minicomputer system, IBM PC-compatible single-user system
Group Size Range:	1 to 30-plus

Suggested Group Size: All are suggested; system is customized to group size

Applications: Accounts payable, appointment scheduling/recall, billing/AR, chart tracking, clinical applications, collections, demographics, electronic claims, fixed assets, general ledger, hospital–physician link, hospital tracking, income distribution, inventory/purchasing, management reporting, medical records, multiple payer privileges, patient registration and history, payroll, physician productivity, prepaid/HMO reporting, spreadsheets, word processing

General Computer Corporation
Address: 2045 Midway Drive, Twinsburg, OH 44087
Phone: 800/521-4548
Hardware: Not available
Group Size Range: Not available
Suggested Group Size: Not available
Applications: Practice management system including billing, AR, electronic claims, appointment scheduling, clinical, and pharmacy system applications

Global Health Systems, Inc.
Address: 1701 Research Boulevard, Rockville, MD 20850
Phone: 301/258-9212; 800/882-7777
Hardware: DEC PDP 11 series and VAX, IBM 9370, 4300 and 3000 series, and HP
Group Size Range: 3 to 200-plus
Suggested Group Size: Not available
Applications: Accounts payable, appointment scheduling/recall, billing/AR, chart tracking, clinical applications, collections, demographics, electronic claims, general ledger, hospital–physician link, hospital tracking, income distribution, management reporting, medical records, multiple payer privileges, patient registration and history, physician productivity, prepaid/HMO reporting, prescription tracking, spreadsheets, utilization review, word processing

GPE Health Systems, Inc.

Address:	36 South State Street, Suite 1900, Salt Lake City, UT 84111
Phone:	801/533-3667
Hardware:	IBM System 38, PC
Group Size Range:	Unlimited
Suggested Group Size:	10 or more physicians
Applications:	Accounts payable, appointment scheduling/recall, billing/AR, chart tracking, clinical applications, collections, demographics, electronic claims, fixed assets, forecasting/modeling, general ledger, hospital–physician link, hospital tracking, income distribution, inventory/purchasing, management reporting, medical records, multiple payer privileges, patient registration and history, payroll, personnel management, physician productivity, prepaid/HMO reporting, prescription tracking, spreadsheets, utilization review, word processing

Great Lakes Office Systems, Inc.

Address:	20620 North Park Boulevard, #222, Shaker Heights, OH 44118
Phone:	216/932-6800; 800/356-4997
Hardware:	HP
Group Size Range:	1 to 200
Suggested Group Size:	4 to 30 physicians
Applications:	Accounts payable, appointment scheduling/recall, billing/AR, chart tracking, clinical applications, collections, demographics, electronic claims, fixed assets, forecasting/modeling, general ledger, hospital tracking, income distribution, inventory/purchasing, management reporting, medical records, multiple payer privileges, patient registration and history, payroll, physician productivity, prepaid/HMO reporting, prescription tracking, spreadsheets, utilization review, word processing

Health America Systems, Inc.

Address:	404 North Milwaukee Avenue, Libertyville, IL 60048
Phone:	708/362-3730

Hardware: Altos, NCR, WYSE, IBM
Group Size Range: 99
Suggested Group Size: 30 to 40 providers
Applications: Accounts payable, appointment scheduling/
                             recall, billing/AR, chart tracking, electronic
                             claims, general ledger, medical records,
                             patient registration and history, payroll,
                             physician productivity, word processing

Health Care Data Systems
Address: 5703 Enterprise Parkway, P.O. Box 608,
                             Dewitt, NY 13214
Phone: 315/446-7111; 800/950-7111
Hardware: IBM System 36, DEC
Group Size Range: Not available
Suggested Group Size: Not available
Applications: Group practice management system includ-
                             ing billing, AR, appointment scheduling,
                             and physician–hospital link capabilities

Healthcare Software Systems, Inc.
Address: 2903 Aspen Drive, Suite E, Loveland, CO
                             80538
Phone: 303/663-1967; 314/531-3558; 312/916-1447
Hardware: IBM PC and System 36
Group Size Range: 1 to 60-plus
Suggested Group Size: Depends on hardware
Applications: Accounts payable, appointment scheduling/
                             recall, billing/AR, chart tracking, collections,
                             demographics, electronic claims, general
                             ledger, hospital tracking, income distribution,
                             inventory/purchasing, multiple payer privi-
                             leges, patient registration and history, pay-
                             roll, physician productivity, prepaid/HMO
                             reporting, utilization review, word processing

Health Micro Data Systems
Address: 583 D'Onofrio Drive, Madison, WI 53719
Phone: 608/883-4637
Hardware: IBM PC, XT, AT, PS2 and compatibles
Group Size Range: Hospitals with fewer than 150 beds; nurs-
                             ing homes, clinics
Suggested Group Size: Not available
Applications: Accounts payable, billing/AR, clinical appli-
                             cations, electronic claims, fixed assets,

general ledger, inventory/purchasing, medical records, patient registration and history, payroll, word processing

Health Software, Inc.

Address: 4440 Logan Way, Youngstown, OH 44505
Phone: 216/759-2103
Hardware: WYSE, IBM PC compatibles
Group Size Range: 299
Suggested Group Size: 11 to 30 physicians
Applications: Accounts payable, appointment scheduling/ recall, billing/AR, chart tracking, clinical applications, electronic claims, general ledger, hospital–physician link, hospital tracking, income distribution, inventory/ purchasing, management reporting, medical records, multiple payer privileges, patient registration and history, payroll, personnel management, prepaid/HMO reporting, prescription tracking, spreadsheets, utilization review, word processing

High Technology Software Products, Inc.

Address: 8200 North Classen Boulevard, Suite 104, Oklahoma City, OK 73114
Phone: 405/848-0480
Hardware: IBM PC and compatibles, Apple II
Group Size Range: 1- to 5-physician office for Apple version; 10-physician office for IBM PC version
Suggested Group Size: No optimum size ideal
Applications: Appointment scheduling/recall, billing/AR, patient registration and history

High Tech Provisioners, Inc.

Address: 2444 Times Boulevard, Suite 225, Houston, TX 77005
Phone: 713/522-6739; 800/635-4073
Hardware: Not available
Group Size Range: Not available
Suggested Group Size: Not available
Applications: Billing, office management, insurance claims, collections, appointment scheduling, clinical, and other applications

HWA International

Address:	1694 Shelby Oaks Drive North, Memphis, TN 38134
Phone:	901/388-6120
Hardware:	IBM, Tandem
Group Size Range:	1 to 60 physicians
Suggested Group Size:	60 physicians
Applications:	Accounts payable, appointment scheduling/recall, billing/AR, chart tracking, clinical applications, collections, electronic claims, fixed assets, general ledger, hospital–physician link, hospital tracking, inventory/purchasing, medical records, patient registration and history, payroll, physician productivity, prescription tracking, spreadsheets, utilization review, word processing

IDX Corporation

Address:	888 Commonwealth Avenue, Boston, MA 02215
Phone:	617/566-6800
Hardware:	DEC
Group Size Range:	2 or more providers to an unlimited number of physicians
Suggested Group Size:	Because IDX offers two different systems for both large and small practices, anywhere from two to an unlimited number of physicians can be served.
Applications:	Accounts payable, appointment scheduling/recall, billing/AR, chart tracking, clinical applications, collections, demographics, electronic claims, fixed assets, forecasting/modeling, general ledger, hospital–physician link, hospital tracking, income distribution, inventory/purchasing, management reporting, medical records, multiple payer privileges, patient registration and history, payroll, personnel management, physician productivity, prepaid/HMO reporting, prescription tracking, spreadsheets, utilization review

IDX Corporation/Burlington Systems

Address:	1500 Shelbourne Road, Burlington, VT 05403

Phone: 802/862-1022; 800/468-4411
Hardware: IBM, DEC
Group Size Range: Solo to 30 physicians [FTE/(largest installa-
                           tion is 64 physicians)]
Suggested Group Size: 1 to 30 physicians
Applications: Accounts payable, appointment scheduling/
                           recall, billing/AR, clinical applications, col-
                           lections, demographics, electronic claims,
                           general ledger, hospital–physician link,
                           inventory/purchasing, management report-
                           ing, patient registration and history, payroll,
                           physician productivity, prepaid/HMO
                           reporting, word processing

Info Systems of North Carolina, Inc.
Address: 7510 East Independence Boulevard, Suite
                           100, Charlotte, NC 28227
Phone: 704/535-7180
Hardware: IBM System 36
Group Size Range: 1 to 50
Suggested Group Size: 3 to 15 physicians
Applications: Accounts payable, appointment scheduling/
                           recall, billing/AR, collections, demographics,
                           electronic claims, general ledger, hospital
                           tracking, income distribution, inventory/
                           purchasing, management reporting, patient
                           registration and history

Integrated Medical Systems, Inc.
Address: 15000 West 6th Avenue, Golden, CO 80401
Phone: 303/279-6116; 800/422-2110
Hardware: IBM PC compatibles
Group Size Range: Small to medium
Suggested Group Size: Not available
Applications: Group practice management, billing, clini-
                           cal appointment scheduling and physician
                           link, and other applications

International Micro Systems, Inc.
Address: 4341 Merriam Drive, Overland Park, KS
                           66203
Phone: 913/677-1137; 800/255-6223
Hardware: IBM PC, XT, AT, PS2 and compatibles
Group Size Range: Up to 15
Suggested Group Size: 5 to 10 physicians

Applications: Accounts payable, appointment scheduling/
                                       recall, billing/AR, general ledger, medical
                                       records, multiple payer privileges, patient
                                       registration and history, payroll, physician
                                       productivity

The Iris Health Information Systems Corporation
Address: 5 Science Park, New Haven, CT 06960
Phone: 203/786-5400
Hardware: DEC PDP 1173 and VAX, IBM PC, XT, AT
Group Size Range: Unlimited
Suggested Group Size: Unlimited
Applications: Chart tracking, demographics, forecasting/
                                       modeling, hospital–physician link, hospital
                                       tracking, management reporting, medical
                                       records, multiple payer privileges, physician
                                       productivity, prescription tracking, utiliza-
                                       tion review, word processing

Kettering AMS, Inc.
Address: 2773 Orchard Run Road, Dayton, OH 45449
Phone: 513/435-6135; 800/221-5584
Hardware: Wang VS series, IBM 36 series—PCs 386
                                       microprocessor
Group Size Range: 99 full-time physicians
Suggested Group Size: Low-end, 2 to 3 physicians; high-end, 25 to
                                       35 full-time physicians
Applications: Accounts payable, billing/AR, collections,
                                       demographics, electronic claims, fixed
                                       assets, hospital tracking, income distribu-
                                       tion, management reporting, multiple payer
                                       privileges, payroll, physician productivity

Kiyo Systems, Inc.
Address: Wilsey Tech Group Building, 5 Civic Plaza,
                                       Newport Beach, CA 92660-5915
Phone: 714/759-9405
Hardware: IBM XT, AT, and compatibles, Zicomp,
                                       Third Coast Technologies, WYSE, Qume,
                                       Convergent Technologies
Group Size Range: User definable
Suggested Group Size: User definable
Applications: Billing/AR, clinical applications, electronic
                                       claims, inventory/purchasing, patient regis-
                                       tration and history, personnel management,

prescription tracking, spreadsheets, utilization review, word processing

M. A. Kouche & Associates

Address:	5600 Spring Mountain Road, 207, Las Vegas, NV 89102
Phone:	702/364-0630
Hardware:	IBM System 3X
Group Size Range:	Clinics, physicians' offices, laboratories
Suggested Group Size:	Not available
Applications:	Practice management, billing, appointment scheduling, physician–hospital link, and clinical applications

Lancraft, Inc.

Address:	100 Pinnacle Way, Suite 145, Norcross, GA 30071
Phone:	404/448-7850
Hardware:	Any 80286 or 80386 machines including IBM, Compaq, TeleVideo, WYSE, Sperry, AT&T
Group Size Range:	100-plus
Suggested Group Size:	Not available
Applications:	Clinical applications, demographics, hospital–physician link, hospital tracking, medical records, patient registration and history, physician productivity, prescription tracking, utilization review, word processing

Lanier Business Systems

Address:	2310 Parklake Drive NE, Atlanta, GA 30345
Phone:	404/270-2000
Hardware:	Not available
Group Size Range:	Any size
Suggested Group Size:	Not available
Applications:	Appointment scheduling, hospital–physician link, AR, billing, and clinical applications

LDS, Inc.

Address:	12301 West 106th Street, Overland Park, KS 66215
Phone:	913/492-5700
Hardware:	HP, IBM System 36 and PCs, TI
Group Size Range:	Up to 99 physicians
Suggested Group Size:	Largest practice utilizing REMEDY has 21 physicians

Applications: Billing/AR, collections, electronic claims,
                           management reporting, medical records,
                           patient registration and history, physician
                           productivity, prepaid/HMO reporting

Ledger Systems, Inc.
Address: 865 Laurel Street, San Carlos, CA 94070
Phone: 415/592-6001
Hardware: Altos, WYSE, OKI, IBM compatibles, TI,
                           Toshiba, HP
Group Size Range: 10 physicians
Suggested Group Size: 5 to 10 physicians
Applications: Practice management, billing, AR, chart
                           tracking, appointment scheduling, and
                           other applications

Lenco Laboratories, Inc.
Address: P.O. Box 862, Lynbrook, NY 11563
Phone: 516/599-4871; 516/599-4834
Hardware: IBM AT and clones
Group Size Range: 256 physicians
Suggested Group Size: 1 to 256 physicians
Applications: Practice management, billing, AR, hospital–
                           physician link, appointment scheduling,
                           and other applications

London & Bradley, Inc.
Address: 2310 Far Hills Avenue, #5, Dayton, OH
                           45419
Phone: 513/293-0692
Hardware: IBM, NCR, NEC (MS-DOS and clones),
                           AT&T (UNIX)
Group Size Range: 1 to 34 (presently have)
Suggested Group Size: Not available
Applications: Appointment scheduling/recall, billing/AR,
                           chart tracking, clinical applications, demo-
                           graphics, electronic claims, fixed assets,
                           general ledger, hospital–physician link,
                           hospital tracking, income distribution,
                           inventory/purchasing, management reporting,
                           medical records, multiple payer privileges,
                           patient registration and history, payroll,
                           physician productivity, prepaid/HMO
                           reporting, prescription tracking, spread-
                           sheets, utilization review, word processing

MAI Basic Four, Inc.

Address:	14101 Myford Road, Tustin, CA 92680
Phone:	714/730-3114
Hardware:	MAI Basic Four
Group Size Range:	There is no practical limitation on the number of physicians that can be served (actual maximum 9,999)
Suggested Group Size:	Because of the breadth of the MAI Basic Four product line, all group sizes can be handled equally well
Applications:	Accounts payable, appointment scheduling/recall

Management Science America, Inc.

Address:	3445 Peachtree Road NE, Atlanta, GA 30326
Phone:	404/239-2000
Hardware:	IBM 370XXX, 30XX, 43XX, 9370; Unisys 1100, 2200, V, A, 29XX, 39XX, 49XX, 59XX, 7XXX; Honeywell DPS8, DPS88, DPS90
Group Size Range:	Medium to large hospitals
Suggested Group Size:	Medium to large hospitals
Applications:	Accounts payable, billing/AR, fixed assets, forecasting/modeling, general ledger, inventory/purchasing, management reporting, payroll, personnel management

Marca Medical Office Systems

Address:	5438 South Harper Avenue, Chicago, IL 60615-5535
Phone:	312/684-4300
Hardware:	HP
Group Size Range:	9,999
Suggested Group Size:	3 to 5 physicians in partnership or group practice
Applications:	Accounts payable, appointment scheduling/recall, billing/AR, demographics, electronic claims, general ledger, management reporting, patient registration and history, payroll, physician productivity, prepaid/HMO reporting, word processing

M.D.P., Inc.

Address:	6825 East Tennessee Avenue, Denver, CO 80224

Phone: 303/320-0497
Hardware: UNIX OS compatibles
Group Size Range: Not available
Suggested Group Size: Not available
Applications: Physician office management, billing, clini-
                          cal, ECG analysis, medical records, and
                          appointment scheduling

Medfax Corporation

Address: South Lake Office Park, Tega Cay Road,
                          Fort Mill, SC 29715
Phone: 803/548-1502
Hardware: NCR, Point 4, 286 and 386 processors
Group Size Range: 1 to 1,000
Suggested Group Size: 1 to 80
Applications: Accounts payable, appointment scheduling/
                          recall, billing/AR, chart tracking, clinical
                          applications, collections, demographics,
                          electronic claims, fixed assets, general
                          ledger, hospital tracking, income distribu-
                          tion, inventory/purchasing, management
                          reporting, medical records, multiple payer
                          privileges, patient registration and history,
                          payroll, physician productivity, prepaid/
                          HMO reporting, prescription tracking, word
                          processing

Medical Accounts Management Service

Address: 14L World's Fair Drive, Somerset, NJ 08873
Phone: 201/539-3880; 800/232-9990
Hardware: IBM PC, XT, System 36, 38
Group Size Range: Not available
Suggested Group Size: Not available
Applications: Billing, AR, collections, electronic claims,
                          appointment scheduling, physician–hospital
                          link, and clinical applications

Medical Computer Management, Inc.

Address: 10810 Forman Drive, Suite 310, Omaha, NE
                          68154
Phone: 402/330-6660
Hardware: Not available
Group Size Range: Not available
Suggested Group Size: Not available

Applications: AR, insurance processing, EMC, medical records, general ledger, accounts payable, payroll, word processing

Medical Data Systems
(Division of General Computer Corporation)
Address: 2045 Midway Drive, Twinsburg, OH 44087
Phone: 216/234-5424; 800/521-4548
Hardware: Not available
Group Size Range: Not available
Suggested Group Size: Not available
Applications: Management system, billing, electronic claims, HMO, PPO, patient recall, medical records, and other applications

Medical Digital Technologies, Inc.
Address: 6901 Canby Avenue, Suite 107, Reseda, CA 91335
Phone: 818/344-8915
Hardware: Alpha Micro and IBM AT compatibles
Group Size Range: 1 to 255
Suggested Group Size: 10 to 200 physicians
Applications: Accounts payable, appointment scheduling/ recall, billing/AR, chart tracking, clinical applications, collections, demographics, electronic claims, general ledger, income distribution, inventory/purchasing, management reporting, medical records, multiple payer privileges, patient registration and history, payroll, physician productivity, prepaid/HMO reporting, prescription tracking, spreadsheets, utilization review, word processing

Medical Group Systems, Inc.
Address: 8730 King George Drive, Suite 104, Dallas, TX 75235
Phone: 214/631-1190
Hardware: IBM System 36, 38
Group Size Range: 1 to 300 physicians
Suggested Group Size: 100 physicians
Applications: Accounts payable, appointment scheduling/ recall, billing/AR, chart tracking, collections, demographics, electronic claims, general ledger, income distribution, management

reporting, patient registration and history,
payroll, physician productivity, prepaid/
HMO reporting, spreadsheets, word
processing

Medical Management Services

Address: 1505 7th Street, Moline, IL 61265-2992
Phone: 309/762-0973
Hardware: None—recommend hardware
Group Size Range: Up to 100 physicians
Suggested Group Size: 50 physicians
Applications: Accounts payable, appointment scheduling/
                          recall, billing/AR, collections, demographics,
                          electronic claims, fixed assets, general
                          ledger, hospital physician link, hospital
                          tracking, income distribution, inventory/
                          purchasing, management reporting, medical
                          records, multiple payer privileges, patient
                          registration and history, payroll, physician
                          productivity, prepaid/HMO reporting, utili-
                          zation review

Medical Office Services, Inc.

Address: 415 West Golf Road, Suite 16, Arlington
                          Heights, IL 60005
Phone: 708/952-3600; 800/323-6671
Hardware: NCR, Altos
Group Size Range: 1 to 100 physicians
Suggested Group Size: Not available
Applications: Financial, patient tracking, patient recall,
                          appointment scheduling, and other appli-
                          cations

Medical Systems, Inc.

Address: 301 Edgewater Place, Suite 300, Wakefield,
                          MA 01880
Phone: 617/245-8944
Hardware: DEC, Unisys, HP, Data General, IBM PC
Group Size Range: 10 to 250 physicians
Suggested Group Size: 10 to 250 physicians
Applications: Accounts payable, appointment scheduling/
                          recall, billing/AR, chart tracking, clinical
                          applications, collections, demographics,
                          electronic claims, fixed assets, forecasting/
                          modeling, general ledger, hospital–physician

link, hospital tracking, income distribution, inventory/purchasing, management reporting, medical records, multiple payer privileges, patient registration and history, physician productivity, prepaid/HMO reporting, prescription tracking, spreadsheets, utilization review, word processing

Medical Systems Support, Inc.

Address:	2301 Moody Parkway, Suite 1, Moody, AL 35004
Phone:	205/699-1080; 800/633-2778
Hardware:	Not available
Group Size Range:	Solo, family, or multipractice
Suggested Group Size:	Not available
Applications:	Billing, clinical, management reporting

Medic Computer Systems
(Subsidiary of Emhart Corporation)

Address:	8601 Six Forks Road, Suite 300, Raleigh, NC 27615
Phone:	919/847-8102
Hardware:	TI 1000 series and IBM PC AT compatibles
Group Size Range:	3 to 10; 10 to 50
Suggested Group Size:	Hardware dependent
Applications:	AR, collections, appointment scheduling, check refunds, history, demographics, electronic claims, medical records, insurance tracking, physician–hospital link

Medicomp of Virginia, Inc.

Address:	9526-A Lee Highway, Fairfax, VA 22031
Phone:	703/591-0914
Hardware:	IBM Series 1 and most computers running UNIX
Group Size Range:	10,000
Suggested Group Size:	20 to 10,000
Applications:	Accounts payable, appointment scheduling/recall, billing/AR, clinical applications, collections, demographics, hospital–physician link, hospital tracking, management reporting, medical records, patient registration and history, personnel management, physician productivity, prepaid/HMO reporting, utilization review, word processing

MegaWest Systems, Inc.

Address:	345 Bearcat Drive, Salt Lake City, UT 84115
Phone:	801/487-0788
Hardware:	General Automation, Fujitsu, Pick OS compatibles
Group Size Range:	Solo through large multispecialty clinics
Suggested Group Size:	Unlimited
Applications:	Accounts payable, appointment scheduling/ recall, billing/AR, clinical applications, collections, electronic claims, fixed assets, income distribution, management reporting, medical records, multiple payer privileges, patient registration and history, payroll, physician productivity, prepaid/HMO reporting, spreadsheets, word processing

MHA Software Services, Inc.

Address:	735 North 120th Street, Omaha, NE 68154
Phone:	402/493-0690
Hardware:	IBM System 36, PC
Group Size Range:	1 to 500,000 active accounts
Suggested Group Size:	Not available
Applications:	Appointment scheduling/recall, billing/AR, collections, demographics, electronic claims, management reporting, medical records, multiple payer privileges, patient registration and history, physician productivity, word processing

Mid-America Business Computers, Inc.

Address:	10705 Barkley, Overland Park, KS 66211-1152
Phone:	913/642-6222
Hardware:	Data General, DEC, IBM PC, NCR, Unisys
Group Size Range:	1 to 1,000 full-time physicians (depends on hardware capacity)
Suggested Group Size:	System can function optimally for any size.
Applications:	Accounts payable, appointment scheduling/ recall, billing/AR, chart tracking, collections, demographics, electronic claims, fixed assets, hospital–physician link, hospital tracking, income distribution, inventory/purchasing, management reporting, multiple payer privileges, patient registration and history, payroll, physician productivity, prepaid/HMO reporting, spreadsheets, word processing

Millard-Wayne, Incorporated
Address: 8100 Roswell Road, Atlanta, GA 30350
Phone: 404/395-7222
Hardware: IBM PS/2, mid-range hardware
Group Size Range: Group clinic and medical center
Suggested Group Size: Not available
Applications: Billing, clinical, appointment scheduling, hospital–physician link

MOS, Inc.
Address: 415 West Golf Road, #16, Arlington Heights, IL 60005
Phone: 708/952-3600; 800/323-6771
Hardware: NCR–CIES
Group Size Range: 70 to 75 physicians
Suggested Group Size: 3 to 20 physicians
Applications: Not available

Multi-Data Systems, Inc.
Address: 7038 Bandera, San Antonio, TX 78238
Phone: 512/684-2983
Hardware: IBM microcomputer compatibles, Okidata, Everex, ACER, WYSE
Group Size Range: Up to 20 physicians in up to 10 locations
Suggested Group Size: 1 to 4 physicians
Applications: Appointment scheduling/recall, billing/AR, chart tracking, clinical applications, collections, demographics, electronic claims, general ledger, hospital tracking, income distribution, management reporting, medical records, multiple payer privileges, patient registration and history, personnel management, physician productivity, prepaid/HMO reporting, prescription tracking, utilization review, word processing

National Medical Computer Services (Subsidiary of the Reynolds and Reynolds Company)
Address: 8928 Terman Court, San Diego, CA 92121
Phone: 619/566-5800; 800/582-6474
Hardware: IBM System 36, models 5360, 5362, 5364, PC, AT
Group Size Range: Depends on system and configuration
Suggested Group Size: Depends on system and configuration

Applications: Appointment scheduling/recall, billing/AR,
                           collections, demographics, income distribu-
                           tion, management reporting, medical
                           records, payroll, personnel management,
                           word processing

National Medical Services, Inc.
Address: 5397 Summerwood Court, Frederick, MD
                           21701
Phone: 301/473-5688
Hardware: Micro based
Group Size Range: Physicians' offices and clinics
Suggested Group Size: Not available
Applications: Billing, appointment scheduling, clinical
                           and hospital–physician links

Occidental Computer Systems, Inc.
Address: 8100 Balboa Boulevard, Van Nuys, CA 91406
Phone: 818/786-9920; 818/712-9011
Hardware: IBM PC compatibles, System 36, 38, main-
                           frames, and HP 3000
Group Size Range: Not available
Suggested Group Size: Not available
Applications: Billing, appointment scheduling, clinical,
                           hospital–physician link, and other
                           applications

Orbis Systems, Inc.
Address: 4039-L Medical Center Drive, McHenry, IL
                           60050
Phone: 815/344-0400
Hardware: Not available
Group Size Range: Not available
Suggested Group Size: Not available
Applications: Physician office management, laboratory,
                           pathology, medical records, pharmacy,
                           medical HMO

OR-D Medical Management Systems
Address: 1414 Brace Road, Cherry Hill, NJ 08034
Phone: 609/795-8300; 800/722-ORD1
Hardware: IBM, Apple, and compatibles
Group Size Range: 16
Suggested Group Size: 16 physicians

Applications: Accounts payable, appointment scheduling/ recall, billing/AR, chart tracking, collections, electronic claims, fixed assets, forecasting/ modeling, hospital–physician link, hospital tracking, income distribution, management reporting, medical records, multiple payer privileges, patient registration and history, physician productivity, prepaid/HMO reporting, prescription tracking, spreadsheets, word processing

Pacific MedSoft, Inc.

Address:	P.O. Box 7049, Tahoe City, CA 95730
Phone:	916/583-2994
Hardware:	IBM compatibles, LANs, SCO Xenix System V
Group Size Range:	99
Suggested Group Size:	1 to 15 physicians
Applications:	Accounts payable, appointment scheduling/ recall, billing/AR, clinical applications, collections, demographics, electronic claims, fixed assets, general ledger, hospital–physician link, hospital tracking, income distribution, inventory/purchasing, management reporting, multiple payer privileges, patient registration and history, personnel management, physician productivity, prepaid/HMO reporting, spreadsheets

PC Specialties

Address:	1040 East Chapman Avenue, Suite A, Orange, CA 92666
Phone:	714/771-3560
Hardware:	Not available
Group Size Range:	Single to multiuser practices
Suggested Group Size:	Not available
Applications:	Billing, clinical, appointment scheduling, hospital–physician link

Pearl Systems Company

Address:	81 Great Valley Parkway, Suite 500, Malvern, PA 19355
Phone:	215/647-2210
Hardware:	HP
Group Size Range:	20
Suggested Group Size:	20 physicians

Applications: Appointment scheduling/recall, billing/AR,
                           electronic claims, income distribution,
                           management reporting, medical records,
                           multiple payer privileges, patient registra-
                           tion and history, payroll, spreadsheets,
                           word processing

Physician Computer Network, Inc.
Address: 225 Christiani Street, Cranford, NJ 07016
Phone: 201/276-1144; 800/221-1476
Hardware: Not available
Group Size Range: Not available
Suggested Group Size: Not available
Applications: Billing, clinical, appointment scheduling,
                           and other applications

Physician Micro Systems, Inc.
Address: 2033 Sixth Avenue, Suite 707, Seattle, WA
                           98121
Phone: 206/441-8490
Hardware: IBM PC compatibles
Group Size Range: Single practice to multiuser
Suggested Group Size: Not available
Applications: Billing, medical records, appointment
                           scheduling, and medical dictation

Physicians' Computer Systems, Inc.
Address: 1313 Gateway Drive, Suite 1014, Melbourne,
                           FL 32901
Phone: 407/984-8680; 800/476-5122
Hardware: IBM PC compatibles
Group Size Range: Not available
Suggested Group Size: Not available
Applications: Billing, clinical, appointment scheduling,
                           and other applications

Physicians' Office Computer
Address: 1240 Kona Drive, Compton, CA 90220
Phone: 213/603-0555
Hardware: Altos, IBM, to local Los Angeles clients
Group Size Range: Up to 99
Suggested Group Size: Hardware dependent
Applications: Accounts payable, appointment scheduling/
                           recall, billing/AR, clinical applications, elec-
                           tronic claims, management reporting, medi-
                           cal records, patient registration and history

Polk County Clinic

Address:	220 North State, Box 197, Osceola, NE 68651
Phone:	402/747-2411
Hardware:	IBM PC compatibles, Tandy
Group Size Range:	Unlimited
Suggested Group Size:	5 physicians
Applications:	Accounts payable, appointment scheduling/ recall, billing/AR, collections, general ledger, income distribution, management reporting, multiple payer privileges, payroll, physician productivity

Poorman-Douglas Corporation

Address:	1325 Southwest Custer Drive, Portland, OR 97219
Phone:	503/245-5555; 800/547-4407
Hardware:	TI business system minicomputers, series 1000 supermicro computers
Group Size Range:	Ledger solution product, 3 to 12 physicians; Med 990 product, 10 to 100 physicians
Suggested Group Size:	3 to 8 physicians on ledger solution, 20 to 50 on Med 990
Applications:	Accounts payable, appointment scheduling/ recall, billing/AR, chart tracking, clinical applications, collections, demographics, electronic claims, general ledger, hospital–physician link, income distribution, management reporting, medical records, multiple payer privileges, patient registration and history, payroll, physician productivity, prepaid/HMO reporting, prescription tracking, spreadsheets, utilization review, word processing

Professional Software Solutions, Inc.

Address:	2718 Southwest Kelly, Suite D, Portland, OR 97201
Phone:	503/221-1552
Hardware:	IBM compatibles
Group Size Range:	Not available
Suggested Group Size:	Not available
Applications:	AR, billing, patient recall, appointment scheduling, referrals, source analysis, Report Write, forms, and electronic claims

Provider Automated Services, Incorporated

Address: 8659 Baypine Road, Suite 200, Jacksonville,
                            FL 32216-7513
Phone: 904/739-6700; 800/334-4916
Hardware: IBM, TI, Altos
Group Size Range: Solo to large groups
Suggested Group Size: Not available
Applications: AR, billing, clinical, appointment
                            scheduling

PRx, Inc.

Address: 43 Bradford Street, Concord, MA 01742
Phone: 508/369-3566
Hardware: IBM PC, mainframe, DEC VAX
Group Size Range: Solo practice to large clinics
Suggested Group Size: Not available
Applications: Billing, appointment scheduling, medical
                            records, management reporting

PSI-MED Corporation

Address: 1221 East Dye Road, Suite 240, Santa Ana,
                            CA 92705
Phone: 714/979-7653
Hardware: HP 3000
Group Size Range: Most installations fall within the 6- to
                            50-physician range
Suggested Group Size: 100 full-time physicians
Applications: Appointment scheduling/recall, billing/AR,
                            collections, demographics, hospital tracking,
                            income distribution, inventory/purchasing,
                            management reporting, medical records,
                            patient registration and history, word
                            processing

Pundsack Computer Services

Address: P.O. Box 1162, Rhinelander, WI 54501
Phone: 715/369-4020
Hardware: IBM AT, PS2 and compatibles, Altos, AT&T
Group Size Range: 200 physicians
Suggested Group Size: 5 to 75 physicians
Applications: Accounts payable, fixed assets, forecasting/
                            modeling, general ledger, income distribu-
                            tion, management reporting, payroll, per-
                            sonnel management, physician productivity,
                            spreadsheets, word processing

Q. S., Inc.

Address:	P.O. Box 847, NCNB Plaza, Suite 1106, Greenville, SC 29602
Phone:	803/232-2666
Hardware:	Prime computers, IBM PC compatibles, mainframes
Group Size Range:	1 to 999
Suggested Group Size:	5 to 6 physicians
Applications:	Appointment scheduling/recall, billing/AR, chart tracking, clinical applications, demographics, electronic claims, fixed assets, forecasting/modeling, general ledger, inventory/purchasing, management reporting, medical records, multiple payer privileges, patient registration and history, payroll, personnel management, prescription tracking

Quality Medical Solutions, Inc.

Address:	60 Commerce Way, Hackensack, NJ 07601
Phone:	201/488-1020; 800/227-2360
Hardware:	IBM, Compaq, DEC
Group Size Range:	Solo to multiphysician
Suggested Group Size:	Not available
Applications:	AR, practice management, appointment scheduling, accounting, word processing, medical records, electronic claims

Quality Systems, Inc. (QSI)

Address:	17822 East 17th Street, Tustin, CA 92680
Phone:	800/854-3433
Hardware:	Quality Systems, Inc.
Group Size Range:	1 to 1,000
Suggested Group Size:	3 to 50 physicians
Applications:	Accounts payable, appointment scheduling/recall, billing/AR, chart tracking, clinical applications, collections, demographics, electronic claims, fixed assets, forecasting/modeling, general ledger, hospital tracking, income distribution, inventory/purchasing, management reporting, medical records, multiple payer privileges, patient registration and history, payroll, personnel management, physician productivity, prepaid/HMO reporting, prescription tracking, spreadsheets, word processing

The Sachs Group

Address:	1800 Sherman Avenue, Evanston, IL 60201
Phone:	708/492-7526
Hardware:	IBM, Compaq, Unisys
Group Size Range:	Any size
Suggested Group Size:	No size is better than any other
Applications:	Demographics, forecasting/modeling

SCI/Fortune Systems

Address:	2000 Ringwood Avenue, San Jose, CA 95131
Phone:	408/943-6200
Hardware:	UNIX-based microcomputers
Group Size Range:	Small and large physicians' offices, clinics
Suggested Group Size:	Not available
Applications:	Billing, clinical, appointment scheduling, hospital–physician link, and other applications

Science Dynamics Corporation

Address:	2140 West 190th Street, Torrance, CA 90504
Phone:	213/320-1101; 800/421-2181
Hardware:	DEC VAX, Micro VAX, developing HP 3000 and IBM AS 400
Group Size Range:	3 to 100
Suggested Group Size:	Hardware dependent
Applications:	AR, billing, registration, collection management, HMO and PPO management, utilization review, cash posting, referral tracking, sequential billing, Report Writer, patient appointment scheduling, claims tracking, and management reports

Seako, Inc.

Address:	517 Beacon Parkway West, Birmingham, AL 35209
Phone:	205/945-8200; 800/255-0869
Hardware:	IBM, NEC
Group Size Range:	Not available
Suggested Group Size:	Not available
Applications:	Billing, clinical, appointment scheduling, hospital–physician link

Shebele, Inc.

Address:	P.O. Box 816, Havertown, PA 19038
Phone:	215/446-2449

Hardware: IBM PC, AT, compatibles, NCR, DEC
Group Size Range: Small to large
Suggested Group Size: Not available
Applications: Billing, clinical, appointment scheduling

SMS

Address: 51 Valley Stream Parkway, Malvern, PA 19355
Phone: 215/296-6300
Hardware: IBM, DEC, Telex, Netlink, S-36
Group Size Range: 400-plus
Suggested Group Size: 3 to 300 physicians
Applications: Practice management, accounts payable, appointment scheduling/recall, billing/AR, chart tracking, clinical applications, collections, demographics, electronic claims, general ledger, hospital–physician link, hospital tracking, income distribution, inventory, purchasing, management reporting, medical records, multiple payer privileges, patient registration and history, payroll, personnel management, physician productivity, prepaid/HMO reporting, spreadsheets, utilization review, word processing

Software Associates, Inc.

Address: 201 Benton Avenue, Linthicum, MD 21090
Phone: 301/859-0002
Hardware: IBM System 36, all models
Group Size Range: 1 to 99
Suggested Group Size: More than 2 physicians
Applications: Accounts payable, appointment scheduling/recall, billing/AR, collections, demographics, electronic claims, general ledger, inventory/purchasing, management reporting, medical records, patient registration and history, payroll, physician productivity, prepaid/HMO reporting

Southern Software Systems, Inc.

Address: 1644 Shadow Moss, Germantown, TN 38138
Phone: 901/365-7550
Hardware: Data General

Group Size Range: Up to 100
Suggested Group Size: 2 to 20 physicians
Applications: Accounts payable, appointment scheduling/
                         recall, billing/AR, chart tracking, collections,
                         demographics, electronic claims, fixed
                         assets, general ledger, hospital tracking,
                         income distribution, inventory/purchasing,
                         management reporting, medical records,
                         multiple payer privileges, patient registra-
                         tion and history, payroll, personnel
                         management, physician productivity,
                         prepaid/HMO reporting, prescription track-
                         ing, spreadsheets, utilization review, word
                         processing

SSM Data Center
Address: 7980 Clayton Road, Suite 401, St. Louis,
                         MO 63117
Phone: 314/647-9044
Hardware: Not available
Group Size Range: Not available
Suggested Group Size: Not available
Applications: Billing, clinical

Stradford Healthcare Systems, Inc.
Address: 840 Mitten Road, Burlingame, CA 94010
Phone: 415/692-7970
Hardware: Alpha Micro CPU
Group Size Range: No limit
Suggested Group Size: 1 to 40 physicians
Applications: Appointment scheduling/recall, billing/AR,
                         collections, demographics, electronic claims,
                         income distribution, management report-
                         ing, multiple payer privileges, patient regis-
                         tration and history, payroll, physician
                         productivity, word processing

STARx Technologies
Address: 1201 Flower Street, Bakersfield, CA 93305
Phone: 805/324-6041
Hardware: IBM and compatibles, NCR, Altos, Apple,
                         AT&T, most Unix and Xenix based CPUs
Group Size Range: Unlimited
Suggested Group Size: 1 to 500 physicians

Applications: Accounts payable, appointment scheduling/ recall, billing/AR, chart tracking, collections, demographics, electronic claims, fixed assets, general ledger, hospital–physician link, hospital tracking, income distribution, inventory/purchasing, management reporting, medical records, multiple payer privileges, patient registration and history, payroll, personnel management, physician productivity, prepaid/HMO reporting, prescription tracking, spreadsheets, utilization review, word processing

Systems Architecture

Address:	370 West Camino Gardens Boulevard, Boca Raton, FL 33432
Phone:	407/392-9800; 800/553-0777
Hardware:	DEC VAX, IBM PC, Novell, LAN
Group Size Range:	Not available
Suggested Group Size:	Not available
Applications:	Billing, electronic claims, appointment scheduling, HMO, PPO, IPA applications

Systems Plus, Inc.

Address:	500 Clyde Avenue, Mountain View, CA 94043
Phone:	415/969-7047; 800/222-7701
Hardware:	Not available
Group Size Range:	1 to 999 physicians
Suggested Group Size:	Not available
Applications:	Billing, practice management, reporting, and clinical and appointment scheduling

Tampa Data Services, Inc.

Address:	1338 Woodcrest Avenue, Clearwater, FL 34616
Phone:	813/461-4486
Hardware:	Data General Eclipse and MV series minicomputers
Group Size Range:	Small to large
Suggested Group Size:	Not available
Applications:	Patient billing, clinical reporting, insurance processing, financial management, and patient appointment scheduling

Terrano Corporation
Address: 245 South 84th Street, Suite 215, Lincoln,
                          NE 68510
Phone: 402/483-7831
Hardware: Prime 50 series, 32-bit super minicomputers
Group Size Range: Unlimited
Suggested Group Size: Not available
Applications: Billing/AR, electronic claims, general ledger,
                          word processing

Trinity Computing Systems, Inc.
Address: 11 Greenway Plaza, Suite 12, Houston, TX
                          77046
Phone: 713/621-6911; 800/231-2445
Hardware: IBM PC, XT, AT, PS2
Group Size Range: Hospital systems—200 users (stations)
Suggested Group Size: Not available
Applications: Patient registration and history

Unisys Healthcare Systems
Address: 2101-W Rexford Road, Charlotte, NC 28211
Phone: 704/362-9600
Hardware: Unisys B2X, B3X, XE500 series
Group Size Range: Not dependent on number of physicians—
                          dependent on practice patient volume
Suggested Group Size: Not dependent on number of physicians—
                          dependent on practice patient volume
Applications: Accounts payable, appointment scheduling/
                          recall, billing/AR, chart tracking, electronic
                          claims, forecasting/modeling, general ledger,
                          hospital–physician link, inventory/purchasing,
                          medical records, multiple payer privileges,
                          patient registration and history, payroll,
                          physician productivity, prepaid/HMO
                          reporting, spreadsheets, word processing

Wallaby Software Corporation
Address: 10 Industrial Avenue, Mahway, NJ 07430
Phone: 201/934-9333
Hardware: AT&T, Altos, Fortune, IBM and compatibles,
                          and NCR
Group Size Range: Number of physicians is dependent on
                          hardware selected; restrictions do not exist.
Suggested Group Size: Number of physicians is dependent on
                          hardware selected; restrictions do not exist.

Applications: Appointment scheduling/recall, billing/AR, chart tracking, collections, demographics, electronic claims, management reporting, medical records, multiple payer privileges, patient registration and history, physician productivity, prepaid/HMO reporting, prescription tracking, utilization review

Westland Medical Systems

Address:	23901 Calabasas Road, Suite 1064, Calabasas, CA 91302
Phone:	818/992-0081; 800/423-5880
Hardware:	HP series 260 minicomputer
Group Size Range:	1 to 25
Suggested Group Size:	3 to 15 physicians
Applications:	Accounts payable, appointment scheduling/recall, billing/AR, collections, demographics, electronic claims, general ledger, hospital tracking, management reporting, medical records, multiple payer privileges, patient registration and history, payroll, physician productivity, prepaid/HMO reporting, word processing

Westland Software House, Inc.

Address:	20847 Sherman Way 300, Canoga Park, CA 91306
Phone:	818/992-0081; 800/423-5880
Hardware:	Not available
Group Size Range:	Not available
Suggested Group Size:	Not available
Applications:	Billing, medical records, and appointment scheduling

Wismer * Martin

Address:	North 12828 Newport Highway, Spokane, WA 99218
Phone:	509/466-0396; 800/231-7477
Hardware:	IBM PC compatibles, Novell LAN
Group Size Range:	Single to multiuser
Suggested Group Size:	Not available
Applications:	Billing, accounts management, electronic claims processing, appointment scheduling, hospital–physician link

Zybex, Inc.

Address:	10655 Roselle Street, San Diego, CA 92121
Phone:	619/459-2797; 800/328-2299
Hardware:	Alpha Micro
Group Size Range:	Either individual practitioner or groups, IPA groups, and HMOs
Suggested Group Size:	Multiphysician practices
Applications:	Accounts payable, appointment scheduling/recall, billing/AR, chart tracking, collections, demographics, electronic claims, fixed assets, forecasting/modeling, general ledger, hospital–physician link, hospital tracking, income distribution, inventory/purchasing, management reporting, medical records, multiple payer privileges, patient registration and history, payroll, personnel management, physician productivity, prepaid/HMO reporting, prescription tracking, spreadsheets, utilization review, word processing

Appointment Scheduling Vendors

ACPI Ltd., Division of Advanced Institutional Management Software
485 Underhill Boulevard
Syossett, NY 11791-3413
516/496-7700

American Business Computers, Inc.
140 North Highway 227
P.O. Box 936
Clute, TX 77531
409/265-2573; 800/237-5036

Andent, Inc.
1000 North Avenue
Waukegan, IL 60085
708/223-5077

Applied Information Management Sciences, Inc.
2900 DeSoto Street
Monroe, LA 71201
318/323-2467; 800/551-5187

AT&T
100 Southgate Parkway
Morristown, NJ 07960
201/898-8176

CARE Info Systems, Inc.
P.O. Box 11140
Springfield, IL 62791
217/529-0255

C&S Research
210 Goddard Boulevard
King of Prussia, PA 19406
215/265-9118

Central Hospital Computer Services, Inc.
Airport Executive Office
510 Plaza Drive
Suite 300
Atlanta, GA 30349
800/451-6420

Note: This listing was prepared by staff at the Harvard Community Health Plan, Brookline, Massachusetts, and does not in any way represent support for any particular vendors. Some vendors may have been inadvertently omitted. Readers are advised to contact listed firms on an ongoing basis because relevant information may be revised occasionally.

CyCare Systems
4343 E. Camelback Road
Phoenix, AZ 85018
602/952-5300

Database, Inc.
1803A Chapel Hill Road
Durham, NC 27707
919/393-6969

Data Strategies
17150 Via Del Campo
Suite 203
San Diego, CA 92127
619/451-0480

**Dental Data Management
Systems**
23 Northcote Drive
Melville, NY 11747
516/491-7558

Elcomp Systems, Inc.
Foster Plaza VI
681 Anderson Drive
Pittsburgh, PA 15220
412/937-0690; 800/441-8386

Epic Systems Corporation
5609 Medical Circle
Madison, WI 53719
608/271-9000

**Ferranti Health Care
(formerly Pentamation
Enterprises)**
4 North Park Drive
Hunt Valley, MD 21030
301/771-1000

Future Tech
701 Scarboro Road
Suite 2015
Oak Ridge, TN 37830
615/482-2461

Global Health Systems, Inc.
1701 Research Boulevard
Rockville, MD 20850
301/258-9212; 800/882-7777

GTE Health Systems, Inc.
36 South State Street
Suite 1900
Salt Lake City, UT 84111
801/533-3637

Health America Systems, Inc.
404 North Milwaukee Avenue
Libertyville, IL 60048
708/362-3730

**Healthcare Computer
Associates**
587 Bethlehem Pike
Suite 300
Montgomeryville, PA 18936
215/822-7055; 800/441-1498

**Health Data Development
Corporation**
5225 Wilshire Boulevard
Suite 220
Los Angeles, CA 90036
213/670-6800

Healthware, Inc.
5397 Summerwood Court
Frederick, MD 21701
301/473-5688

Hewlett-Packard Company
3000 Minuteman Road
Andover, MA 01810-1085
508/687-1501

ICS Technologies
820 West Gerald Avenue South
Elgin, IL 60120
708/931-1963

IDX
888 Commonwealth Avenue
Boston, MA 02215
617/566-6800

Infomaint, Inc.
5397 Summerwood Court
Frederick, MD 21701
301/473-5779

Inteck, Inc.
720 South Colorado Boulevard
Suite 820
Denver, CO 80222
303/759-5511

Intellectual Software
33A Commerce Drive
Fairfield, CT 06430
203/335-0906

International Micro Systems
4331 Merriam Drive
Overland Park, KS 66203
913/677-1137

K-Comp Systems
535 North Grand Boulevard
Suite 601
Glendale, CA 91203
818/500-7222

Knowledge Data Systems
102 West 500 South
Suite 600
Salt Lake City, UT 84101
801/355-7100

Lanier Business Systems
2310 Parklake Drive NE
Atlanta, GA 30345
404/270-2000

LDS, Inc.
12301 West 106th Street
Suite 200
Overland Park, KS 66215
913/492-5700

Lizcon Computer Systems
431 South 300 East
Suite 105
Salt Lake City, UT 84111
801/532-7193

Medfax, Inc.
Tega Cay Road
South Lake Office Park
Fort Mill, SC 29715
803/548-1502

Medical Data Services Corporation
902 Moorefield Park Drive
Richmond, VA 23236
804/272-2828; 800/445-0209

Medical Information Technology
Meditech Circle
Westwood, MA 02090
617/329-5300

Medical Systems Inc.
301 Edgewater Place
Suite 300
Wakefield, MA 01880
617/245-8944

Medidentic, Inc.
Systems Architecture
460 South Northwest Highway
Park Ridge, IL 60068
708/696-0220

Megalo Software Systems
1 Broadway
Suite 300
Denver, CO 80203
303/778-7165

MegaWest Systems, Inc.
345 Bearcat Drive
Salt Lake City, UT 84115
801/487-0788

Millard Wayne, Inc.
8100 Roswell Road
Suite 200
Atlanta, GA 30350
404/395-7222

MTA Systems
4312 West Genesee Street
Syracuse, NY 13215
315/488-1518

National Computer Systems
5605 Green Circle Drive
Minnetonka, MN 55343
612/933-2800

Physician Micro Systems, Inc.
2033 6th Avenue
Suite 707
Seattle, WA 98121
206/441-8490

PRx Inc.
43 Bradford Street
Concord, MA 01742
508/369-3566

Q. S., Inc.
P.O. Box 847
NCNB Plaza
Suite 1106
Greenville, SC 29602
803/232-2666

Quality Data Systems
Library Lane
Old Lyme, CT 06371
203/434-9275

RUF Corp.
1533 East Spruce
Olathe, KS 66061
913/782-8544

Salcris Systems
3550 Independence Drive
Birmingham, AL 35209
205/871-4200

Scitor Corp.
393 Vintage Park Drive
Suite 140
Foster City, CA 94404
415/570-7700

Shared Medical Systems
51 Valley Stream Parkway
Malvern, PA 19355
215/296-6300

John Snow, Inc.
210 Lincoln Street
Boston, MA 02111
617/482-9485

Software Associates, Inc.
201 Benton Avenue
Linthicum, MD 21090
301/859-0002

Southern Software Systems, Inc.
1644 Shadow Moss
Germantown, TN 38138
901/365-7550

Systemedics, Inc.
P.O. Box 11756
Eugene, OR 97440-3956
503/484-4081

TDS HealthCare Systems Corp.
5887 Glenridge Drive
Atlanta, GA 30328
404/847-5000; 800/241-6055

Texas Processor
8122 Datapoint Drive
Ashford Oaks, Suite 910
San Antonio, TX 78229-3228
512/690-9062

Trax Medical Systems
1800 Century Boulevard NE
Suite 880
Atlanta, GA 30345
404/633-3248

Ultrasoft Inc.
1227 Buschong Drive
Houston, TX 77039
713/449-5145

Wallaby Software Corp.
10 Industrial Avenue
Mahwah, NJ 07430
201/934-9333

Annotated Bibliography

Overview

Austin, C. J. Information technology and the future of health services delivery. *Hospital and Health Services Administration* 34(2):157–65, Summer 1989.

> This article examines the dramatic ways that information technology will influence clinical care, strategic management, and organization of the health care delivery system. Advancements in microprocessors, telecommunications, mass storage of data and images, and input-output devices will be accompanied by increased use of health-related software packages. Standardized patient record formats and coding systems will facilitate system integration and networking of computers. Clinical decision support systems will assist physicians in medical diagnosis and treatment. Computer-enhanced medical imaging and other noninvasive procedures will reduce surgery, patient pain and discomfort, and costs. Computerization will get closer to the patient. Management information and decision support systems will be central to effective management in a highly competitive environment. Information systems will support strategic planning, cost control, productivity enhancements, quality improvements, and evaluation of products and services.

Daniels, M. A., Lundquist, S. H., and Simons, P. A. Patient care information systems in a diversified environment. *Topics in Health Care Financing* 14(2):35–41, Winter 1987.

> The growth of the ambulatory care/diversified services environment has created new information requirements for health care institutions.

Information must be accessible to a much larger number of providers practicing in a larger number of settings. Some of these settings may be in the hospital, whereas others may be in remote locations throughout the hospital's service area, including physicians' offices. Certain information management requirements are particular to this expanded environment. Integration is important to ensure accuracy, accessibility, and cost-effectiveness. The information system must be able to serve multiple users across multiple entities. Finally, the hospital should be aware of how the information needs in this new environment are changing key areas such as nursing, pharmacy, and laboratory. This article discusses the various needs associated with managing information in a new diversified environment specifically through the use of several case studies.

Dorenfest, S. I. Charting the course of hospital automation. *Healthcare Executive* 3(1):15–17, Jan.–Feb. 1988.

The newer emerging computer applications for use in the HMO/PPO, home health care, and physician office environments are growing very rapidly. Along with consulting, expenditures for these applications have increased from slightly more than 5 percent of total hospital computer expenditures in 1979 ($48 million) to 16.4 percent in 1986 ($525 million). Given these investment patterns, this article proceeds to explore future changes in various computer applications and how these changes will affect hospital computerization. The author specifically examines changes in the areas of patient accounting, patient care, laboratory, and pharmacy information systems. Because microcomputers are both inexpensive and simple to use, computerization has reached almost every department in the hospital. Among the new applications are computer systems that aid in implementing competitive strategies such as diversification. Newer applications discussed include HMO information systems, home health care information systems, hospital–physician links, and cost accounting and productivity measurement systems.

Flanagan, P. Emergency treatment for health care systems. *Computer Decisions* 16(9):43–49, Sept. 1988.

As hospitals find themselves operating in a more cost-conscious and revenue-restrictive environment, they are seeking information systems that enforce cost-containment strategies. That means the costs of hospital care must be monitored and tracked for each procedure, test, meal, and person each day for each bed. As a result, information managers are being charged with building systems that track and report every bed's profit and loss potential at any time. To do so, information services is branching out of its financial enclave and seeking new links between two separate flows of hospital information: patient care information and accounting and billing. This article explores and discusses the new role information systems play in assisting hospitals to manage this new competitive, cost-conscious environment. It examines the emergence of integrated information systems, the critical role the chief information officer plays in this environment, and future applications of new technology in the patient care process. The article also contains a series of discussions with experts in the field and how they view the evolving information systems environment.

McDonald, C. J. Medical information systems of the future. *M.D. Computing* 6(2):82–86, Feb. 1989.

The coming years promise great advances in the storing, recording, and communication of medical data. Handheld computers may make bedside terminals obsolete. CD-ROM's storage capacity will eliminate data retention problems as well as provide for storage images. Physicians should be able to access computers merely through the recognition of voice patterns. Home monitoring equipment that the physician can access by telephone should reduce hospital stays. Computerized decision support, neurocomputing, and cost-cutting through computerization are all concepts at the cutting edge of medical information technology.

McDougall, M. D., Covert, R. P., and Melton, V. B. *Productivity and Performance Management in Health Care Institutions.* Chicago: American Hospital Publishing, 1989.

In today's extremely competitive environment, productivity improvement is everyone's business. Faced with the infinite number of hurdles that hinder operational productivity improvement efforts, hospitals need to employ those tactics that are most effective in their institutions.

Responding to the difficulties facing hospitals today, the contributors to this book have set forth multiple strategies for obtaining excellent performance and high levels of productivity. By adopting such strategies, hospital management can take a more aggressive approach to improving the utilization of human resources, the quality of health care services, and the selection and performance of employees. An example of such a strategy involves improving the utilization of staff through innovations in patient and employee scheduling. Many departments experience distinct fluctuations in work load throughout the shift, day, week, month, or year. By improving the match between staffing patterns and work load, together with minimizing the peak/valley syndrome typically associated with delivering health care services, hospitals can dramatically improve the utilization and productivity of their human resources.

Successful productivity improvement and performance management efforts all have one major common attribute: complete support from top-level administration. Administrators must actively champion strategies that enable management and staff to perform their duties most effectively and efficiently. Without complete support from top-level management, the expected benefits from a productivity improvement effort may be limited. But the effective use of well-thought-out strategies can improve an organization's bottom line, quality of care, and its competitive advantage over other institutions.

Matson, T. A. *Restructuring for Ambulatory Care: A Guide to Reorganization.* Chicago: American Hospital Publishing, 1990.

Providers intent on becoming significant players in ambulatory care delivery face many diverse and complex challenges—not the least of which is to be both competitively structured and financially viable. Key issues and concerns for those seeking an edge in ambulatory service delivery include understanding the complexities of the various ambulatory care service segments; weighing the value of possible service options and the need for integration; and addressing the management, structural, technological, and operational implications of an ambulatory care strategy.

Overall, a new philosophy must be embraced to effectively meet the demands of ambulatory care services. Programs must be organizationally structured for success and must receive top priority from the board of trustees and senior management. State-of-the-art systems must be in place to monitor and carry out decision making in fast-paced situations. Managers will have to acquire the mind-set and actions of entrepreneurs by assuming a true business orientation for all profit and loss decisions; act as innovators to continually seek out new and different approaches to managing resources, personnel, and service offerings; and embrace an aggressive mentality and political astuteness to defend actions and positions.

Matta, K. F. The impact of prospective pricing on the information system in the health care industry. *Journal of Medical Systems* 12(1):57–66, Feb. 1988.

The move from a retrospective payment system (value added) to a prospective payment system (diagnosis related) has not only influenced the health care business but has also changed its information systems requirements. The change in requirements can be attributed both to an increase in data-processing tasks and also to an increase in the need for information to manage the organization more effectively. A survey was administered to capture the response of health care institutions, in the area of information systems, to the prospective payment system. The survey results indicate that the majority of health care institutions have responded by increasing their information resources, both in terms of hardware and software, and have moved to integrate the medical and financial data. In addition, the role of the information system has changed from a cost accounting system to one intended to provide a competitive edge in a highly competitive marketing environment.

Pierskalla, W. P., and Woods, D. Computers in hospital management and improvements in patient care—new trends in the United States. *Journal of Medical Systems* 12(6):411–28, Dec. 1988.

The health care delivery system, and more particularly the hospital component of the delivery system, is built on having the appropriate people obtain the appropriate information at the right time in order to deliver the optimal care to the patient. As the health care system becomes more complex, the demand for decision-making uses of information grows exponentially. Information systems have a key role in the delivery of health care in the United States. In combination with decision-based and model-based support systems, information systems contribute to improved decision making, improved quality of patient care, improved productivity, and reduced costs. This article discusses the current state of information systems in hospital management. Decision support systems for the management, administrative, and patient care units of the hospital are described. These decision support systems include market planning, nurse scheduling, and blood screening systems. Trends for future uses of computing in hospital management and patient care are analyzed.

Top hospital CEOs chart future MIS directions. *National Report on Computers and Health* 10(6):4–5, Mar. 6, 1989.

In a survey conducted by the Kennedy Group for the Healthcare Information and Management Systems Society of the American Hospital Association, 50 hospital CEOs were asked to identify the direction they would like their information to take. The key areas included networking (including physician offices), interfacing with diagnostic and clinical equipment, bedside systems to increase productivity, imaging, character and voice recognition, physician and clinical support systems, and decision support systems. According to the study, CEOs agree that incorporating information systems into the corporate strategic plan is essential. Systems should be thought of in terms of systems, not applications. They should be viewed as a corporate resource (an investment), not as competition for corporate resources (an expenditure). Commitment must involve the board, executive management, medical staff, and user departments. Flexibility and change within the department are essential to the success of the information system. Managing and using information systems means achieving measurable benefits in terms of dollars, quality of information and care, or strategic positioning.

System Implementation and Evaluation

Albachten, D. R. Proving return on investment: computerized referral tracking and admissions reconciliation. *Computers in Healthcare* 10(1):3032, 3036, Jan. 1989.

> The idea of physician and health care services referral is as old as hospitals. Nearly every hospital in the country receives calls from potential consumers interested in being directed to a physician or service that can help them address a particular medical need. Patients benefit by having their questions answered, hospitals benefit by building market share in times of shrinking reimbursement, and physicians benefit by having a new source of patients. Since 1983, over 50 percent of the nation's health care facilities have formed physician and health care services referral centers. Some of these referral centers are highly sophisticated computerized systems that enable the consumer referral representative to search and sort through a physician and health services data base to find just the right match. Also, these computer systems can generate followup mailings to the callers and the referred physicians and services to keep the referral service (and thus the sponsoring hospital) in mind. This article provides an overview of the referral system concept including cost of operation, benefits of sponsoring one, and methods of measuring the performance and success of the referral system itself. It also describes the MATCHlink referral system developed by Healthline Systems, a company that provides software to assist in marketing, staff credentialing, and risk evaluation.

Austin, H. Assessing the performance of information technology. *Computers in Healthcare* 9(11):56–58, Nov. 1988.

> A recent study conducted by a research team at the Massachusetts Institute of Technology's Sloan School of Management sought answers to selected questions on information technology. The CEOs were asked about their beliefs and assumptions about information technology. The study found that many CEOs are "less than completely satisfied with the methods used in their organization for assessing performance." One factor contributing to this dissatisfaction

is the lack of communication between the CEO and the CIO (chief information officer) in defining their expectations of the management information system. This lack of communication can also be attributed to the divergent management visions held by either the CIO or the CEO. Because these management visions utilize information technology differently to meet institutional goals, different assessment procedures may be required for each. In the Massachusetts Institute of Technology's survey, seven measurements were selected that were most representative of the CEOs' feelings. The seven selected were (1) productivity, (2) user utility, (3) value chain, (4) competitive performance, (5) business alignment, (6) investment targeting, and (7) management vision. The authors define and describe these seven measurements and conclude with a discussion of their relationship to computing in the health care field.

Lemon, R., and Crudele, J. System integration: tying it all together. *Healthcare Financial Management* 41(6):46–48, 52, 54, June 1987.

Health care organizations' changing priorities have created needs for new information systems, as well as a demand for better integration of existing systems. Ten years ago, data processing concentrated on general and patient accounting, payroll, and accounts payable. Today, automated systems have to be able to gather data from several different systems to help in the added areas of patient care, cost management, and marketing. Making the transition from a manual to a truly integrated system is a gradual process, but one that will realize long-term benefits such as increased system efficiency, improved patient care, and better strategic business support. Before taking this step, health care executives need to know the typical problems that may occur with integration and what factors to consider before developing an integrated system. This article discusses changing processing priorities in the health care environment as they relate to system integration, as well as the benefits of integration.

Mann, G. J. Managers, groups, and people: some considerations in information system change. *Health Care Management Review* 13(4):43–48, Fall 1988.

Implementation of a new management information system is dependent to a great extent on the personnel involved. How well or how poorly those affected by a change in information systems accept and implement it depends on several factors, including (1) the effect of the change on the need satisfaction of the affected personnel, (2) the influence of groups, and (3) the leadership style of those managing the change. This article represents the results of a study to investigate anticipated relationships among the factors of need satisfaction, group influence, leadership style, and individual reaction to information system change. The setting for the study was a large health science center in the southwestern United States that installed a new computer-based financial information system to replace the previous system. Analysis of the findings revealed that strong relationships existed between these items: (1) group norms regarding the new information system and the beliefs and attitudes of the subjects toward the new system, (2) growth needs and individual beliefs and attitudes toward the new information system, and (3) leadership style and intentions to support the change. The article concludes with a series of recommendations that managers should incorporate into the planning and execution of change.

Metzger, J. B., Stevens, J. M., Murphy, M. S., and others. A model for capacity planning of a comprehensive integrated information system for hospitals and clinics. *Journal of Medical Systems* 12(4):231–48, June 1988.

> Appropriate system sizing is essential to ensuring a reasonable computer response time for end users. A model is discussed that describes the type and number of interactions between user terminals and printers and the central processor for a comprehensive, integrated medical information system. The system modeled includes support to inpatient and outpatient order entry and results reporting for clinical services; registration; admission, disposition, and transfer; patient appointing; pharmacy, clinical laboratory, and radiology; medical record management; and electronic messages. Originally developed for use in benchmark testing of comprehensive systems designed for military hospitals and clinics, the model has been generalized to be applicable to other systems and settings. Results are presented for a routine busy day in a large freestanding clinic and a 200-bed teaching hospital providing extensive outpatient services. The model results can be applied to several facets of system planning, including sizing of the central processor and communications network, determining the optimal number of storage and user devices, and fine-tuning the user interface.

Roth, M. D. Computer contracting for ambulatory care providers. *Journal of Ambulatory Care Management* 12(2):67–74, May 1989.

> As the health care delivery system continues to shift certain services to the ambulatory care side of the health care equation, computers will be increasingly used, no doubt, by ambulatory care providers to perform a variety of financial, regulatory, and patient care tasks. Given this fact, ambulatory care providers will need to pay serious heed to the phrase "let the buyer beware" when they contract to purchase extremely expensive and sophisticated computer systems. This

article discusses elements that should be included within a contract in order to safeguard the financial interests of an ambulatory care provider when purchasing a computer system.

Toole, J. E., and Caine, M. E. Laying a foundation for future information systems. *Topics in Health Care Financing* 14(2):17–27, Winter 1987.

Changes in the health care environment dictate changes in the development and implementation of hospital information systems. Faced with an explosion of information needs emanating from the executive suite, hospital data-processing management must respond. As the authors state, the critical success factor in establishing a solid information-processing foundation is proper planning. The integration of the strategic business plan with the strategic information plan provides data-processing management the opportunity to develop a sound transition plan and prevents costly errors by institutions forced into a reactive mode by marketplace events. Successful planning is more than developing an outline of information needs. It involves anticipating technology, making a realistic assessment of current capabilities, properly identifying such resource requirements as costs and labor, and developing a realistic action plan. The article provides a concise summary of selected computerization trends and corresponding strategies.

Benefits of Computerization

Austin, C. J. The leading edge. *Health Progress* 70(9):52–54, Oct. 1989.

Management information systems—essential for strategic planning and management in today's complex health care environment—must be designed in concert with goals and strategies developed at the executive or corporate level. Health care organizations need management information to support four major functions: strategic planning and marketing, resource allocation, performance assessment, and evaluation of products and services. Computer systems fall into three general categories: administrative, clinical, and decision support (management information systems). Management information systems are the least advanced of the three. The need for strategic planning and managerial control in the face of complexity and competition, however, will result in rapid advances. The chief executive officer must be responsible for the following areas to ensure the effective use of information systems: strategic planning, information systems planning, user-driven focus, systems integration, and monitoring of results. Many larger health care organizations have established the position of chief information officer (CIO) to assist in these tasks. The CIO coordinates information systems, telecommunications, management engineering, and office automation.

Brivio, O., and Palasciano, C. Automation in the health sector: a cost-benefit analysis methodology for its applications. *Journal of Clinical Computing* 17(4):99–103, 1989.

> The introduction of information technology in the health care setting answers the needs of an operational nature (typically, it allows a reduction in or limits the expansion of costs relating to the execution of a series of activities of a prevalently administrative nature). It also answers the need for coordination and control of activities and health structures (it allows, for example, access to information required for the latter activity in real time in order to intervene in management situations even while that situation is evolving). It also meets requirements of a strategic nature relating to the quality of the service provided (consider the importance of rapid access to complete and reliable health records) and also for providing new services. This article presents a methodology for evaluating costs and benefits of information technology applications in health care environments. The methodology proposes to provide a support tool for the authorities who have to make decisions in terms of information technology investments. It defines the objectives of the process and delineates the various stages of the process. The reasoning behind the methodology and its objectives is also presented.

Couch, J. B. Proving your worth. *Health Progress* 70(5):58–60, May 1989.

> To attract and retain the technologically sophisticated employees needed to compete in today's global environment, American corporations must provide premium employee health benefit packages. Thus, the corporate sector is increasingly demanding proof of quality and cost-effectiveness in benefit plans. One aid in this effort is clinical performance information systems. These systems can help businesses select for their benefit plans the health care providers that produce the greatest improvement in the health status and productivity of employees or plan subscribers per dollar spent. This is known as medical care value purchasing. The systems also help hospital trustees, executives, and medical staff work together to demonstrate and improve the quality of medical care they provide, known as medical care enhancement. This article illustrates how clinical performance information systems can be used by both purchasers and providers of health care to evaluate their own clinical quality and cost-effectiveness. It also describes six major clinical performance systems presently on the market. Use of these systems will permit hospitals to determine how their clinical performance measures up

to that of their competitors. Their standing will be an important factor in determining whether they are included in employee benefit plans, managed care systems, and other preferred provider arrangements.

Oman, R. C., and Ayers, T. Productivity and benefit-cost analysis for information technology decisions. *Information Management Review* 3(3):31–41, Winter 1988.

Information technology is a growth industry in the United States with billions of dollars in sales. Supporters argue that it dramatically increases productivity; critics say productivity is static while costs increase. There is little agreement among technical experts or among organization bureaucrats about whether information technology is a sound investment for organizations or is cost-effective. Indeed, at the present time, there is consensus only that there is a wide disparity of opinion regarding the efficiency and effectiveness of information technology applications. This article examines a number of useful approaches to help provide the clear analysis necessary for organizations functioning in an increasingly competitive environment. It provides useful information on productivity and economic analysis concepts, approaches to defining productivity, benefit-cost models, and evaluation models.

Walker, H. K. Grady Memorial's integrated database improves speed, accuracy, and cost containment. *Computers in Healthcare* 10(3):36–37, 40, 42, Mar. 1989.

No one at Grady Memorial Hospital in Atlanta, Georgia, knows exactly how many lives THERESA™ has saved since it went on-line in 1983. It is certain that the computerized information system has speeded medical care delivery, improved diagnosis accuracy, and cut costs at the third largest hospital in the United States. Using THERESA , doctors can call up patient records in seconds from any terminal in the hospital's large downtown campus. THERESA integrates radiology and pharmacy information along with medical data into a single, hospitalwide medical record data base. The 1,000-bed hospital, which has 800,000 outpatient visits per year, plans to have all needed information from every patient encounter on-line. This article discusses the benefits of the THERESA system specifically in the areas of clinical diagnosis, administration, research, and education. It also provides an overview on the computer technology used to develop, implement, and use the THERESA system.

Watlington, A. G. Realizing system benefits: one planned step at a time. *Computers in Healthcare* 10(2):32–34, 36, Feb. 1989.

The qualitative benefits of improved access to or more timely capture of information will no longer suffice as justification for the purchase of sophisticated management information systems. New system installations must now offer quantitative benefits such as reduced labor and material costs or improved cash flow. Benefit realization is dependent on the hospital's culture and management's commitment to achieving results. Other key success factors also relate to the organizational climate. This article discusses one hospital's plan for achieving the desired results with the selection of its information system. The hospital is distinct in that management, before selecting a system, identified where it expected to realize benefits. The computer system will be the tool for benefit realization. The article also provides information on scheduling the implementation of the system, benefit realization, and the lessons learned from the planning process.

Information Systems, Quality Assurance, and Productivity

Anderson, J. G., Jay, S. J., and Anderson, M. N. Physician use of HIS impacts quality of care. *U.S. Healthcare* 5(10):41–42, 46, Oct. 1988.

An experimental program was designed to increase physician use of personal order sets (POS) to enter medical orders into a hospital information system (HIS). Data on HIS use and the advantages of using POS were fed back to educationally influential physicians on four experimental services. Ten other hospital services were assigned to a control group. Data from the HIS tapes indicate that a significant increase in POS use on the experimental services (cardiovascular disease, general surgery, obstetrics and gynecology, and orthopedic surgery) resulted from the program. Moreover, results of the study indicate that increased use of POS significantly reduces the number of errors made in order entry. The results of this study also indicate that the recruitment and training of educationally influential physicians is an effective way of increasing the clinical use of medical information systems. It appears that the influence of these physicians extends far beyond their immediate colleagues and can affect physician assistants and unit secretaries.

Anderson, J. G., Benson, D. S., Schweer, H. M., and others. AMBUQUAL: A computer-supported system for the measurement and evaluation of quality in ambulatory care settings. *Journal of Ambulatory Care Management* 12(1):27–37, Feb. 1989.

This article describes AMBUQUAL, a computer-based framework for the measurement and evaluation of quality in ambulatory care settings. The system incorporates ten parameters that describe ambulatory care activities in terms of their relative effects on the health of the patient in ambulatory care settings. Research results indicate that these parameters measure a single dimension of quality. Moreover, the weight assigned to a parameter is a numerical measure of the extent to which the parameter is perceived as affecting the health status of patients. Furthermore, AMBUQUAL can be used in a variety of ambulatory care settings to study the efficacy of quality assurance programs. Besides describing the AMBUQUAL system itself, this article also provides information on current methods of quality assurance, parameters of ambulatory care, and the implications associated with the use of the AMBUQUAL system.

Girard, R. E. Productivity and information systems. *Computers in Health Care* 10(2):26–30, Feb. 1989.

The application of information systems to enhance cash flow, economic viability, and productivity continues to grow. Productivity involves effective management of people, materials, and dollars. Executive management must demonstrate commitment to productivity by listening and responding to ideas of staff and promoting productivity in daily work. Sometimes information systems are mistakenly thought to be increasing productivity because data are being produced more rapidly. However, real productivity will occur only when information systems are designed after a careful examination of the processes and interrelationships involved. Significant productivity benefits can occur by quick access to data and the elimination of paperwork. Advances in combined voice, data, and graphics capabilities are leading to increased data exchange efficiencies.

Other improvements include the ability to link into patient and insurance records from physician offices and hospitals using shared data bases. It should be noted that these improvements do not necessarily mean improved quality. Instead, hospitals must institute quality management projects. The article emphasizes that although information systems provide a dynamic means of improving health care productivity, it is important that hospitals understand the systems and not be manipulated by them.

Hemeon, F. E., III. Productivity, cost accounting, and information systems. *Topics in Health Care Financing* 15(3):55–67, Spring 1989.

Few hospitals have integrated cost accounting and productivity monitoring within their information systems architecture. This may be caused by inadequacies associated with most information systems planning processes. Planning for decision support systems, such as cost accounting and productivity monitoring, often proceeds independently of the host systems, which contain important operational information. As a result, the validity of information becomes questionable. This article discusses the use of cost accounting and productivity monitoring systems in the health care setting, focusing on such issues as the objectives associated with cost accounting and productivity monitoring systems, designing an information system to accommodate the data needs of cost accounting and productivity monitoring, the effective use of labor standards in the budgeting and monitoring process, and the development of a consistent and fully integrated information systems environment.

Michelson, L. D. Utilization review for ambulatory care: eliminating unnecessary care. *Journal of Ambulatory Care Management* 12(4):7–14, Nov. 1989.

To date, utilization review has solely been the domain of the inpatient side of the health care equation. Utilization review has been of little value in enhancing the quality of ambulatory care or in managing the volume of ambulatory care. In fact, the success of utilization review in the inpatient setting is primarily responsible for the increased volume and soaring costs in ambulatory care. With the increasing emphasis on ambulatory care as a cost-effective alternative to inpatient care, health care researchers, policymakers, and administrators are examining the possibilities utilization review has in managing the costs and quality of ambulatory services. The question then becomes: Can utilization review assist in the management of ambulatory care? The principal focus of utilization review— whether and how long a patient should be admitted to a hospital to undergo a procedure—is obviously irrelevant in this context. What is relevant in managing ambulatory care, however, is the much more fundamental question of medical necessity: Is this procedure medically appropriate for this patient at this time? This article explores and attempts to add clarity to these questions by examining the use of appropriateness standards to be used in the outpatient setting. It discusses the challenges associated with the development and implementation of these standards and the application of these standards. It concludes with a discussion on the use of expert systems in defining and managing appropriateness standards of practice guidelines as they relate to both prospective precertification and retrospective review.

Wieners, W. Quality measurement and severity systems: an overview. *Computers in Healthcare* 10(10):27, 29, 31–32, Oct. 1988.

A new market for software systems has emerged as vendors seek to improve clinical information systems and offer methods for measuring health care quality. Four principal forces outside the hospital drive the need for additional data: state data commission mandates, accreditation standards, federal reimbursement, and marketing. The discussion of quality assurance systems focuses on three different but overlapping types. One was derived from generic screening methodologies, one is based primarily on claims data, and another abstracts detailed clinical information from the patient's medical record. The three clinical severity systems discussed are Medis-Groups (Medical Illness Severity Grouping System), APACHE II (Acute Physiology and Chronic Health Evaluation), and CSI (Computerized Severity Index). The author also discusses UB-82 severity systems and various quality assurance products.

Cost Accounting Systems

Baptist, A. J., Saylor, J., and Zerwekh, J. Developing a cost solid base for a cost accounting system. *Healthcare Financial Management* 41(1):42–44, 46, 48, Jan. 1987.

Henry Ford Hospital recently conducted a procedural costing study to determine whether more accurate costs for various institutional procedures could be developed. The hospital conducted the study in two phases. The first phase looked at a specific department; phase two took a broader approach and covered the entire institution. This article examines the department-specific phase, in which the diagnostic radiology department was selected as the participant. The study concluded that by allocating costs to the procedural level using relative value units and feeding this information into the case mix system, departmental costs could be accurately identified.

Gragg, J. H., and Johnson, J. L. Cost accounting: alive and well for the 1990s. *U.S. Healthcare* 6(4):36, 38, 40, Apr. 1989.

Medical College Hospitals (MCH) in Toledo, Ohio, recently implemented the Health Care Microsystem's (HCM) Standard Costing System, a procedure-level, microcomputer-based cost accounting system. Using the system, the hospital was able to identify detailed direct and indirect costs at the procedure level. This was achieved by defining direct standards for labor and other major classes of expense, including labor time and supply items, to perform each procedure. Expense data were obtained by downloading historical files from the mainframe computer. This article reports on MCH's experiences in implementing and using the system. It provides detailed information on how the facility went about collecting the necessary data to define fixed/variable or direct/indirect costs.

It also discusses how the cost information was used in case management reporting and evaluating the resources used in providing patient care services.

Kis, G., and Bodenger, G. Cost management information improves financial performance. *Healthcare Financial Management* 43(5):36, 38, 40, 42, 44, 46, 48, May 1989.

Hospitals continually face the challenge of providing high-quality medical care at competitive prices. Management must determine which services to offer within the context of their hospital's mission while pricing and delivering those services at a reasonable level of profitability. Cost management information can help hospitals improve their financial and operational performance and better address an array of management issues. Improved cost information enables hospitals to price services more competitively, reduce and control operating costs, and upgrade strategic planning efforts. This article evaluates the role cost management information plays in such areas as competitive pricing, cost control, and strategic planning. It details how cost management information can be used to assist hospitals in determining discount and product volume levels, product margins, summary performance information, efficiency variances, and market potential for products and services. Throughout the article, the authors provide detailed charts and graphs that illustrate the statistical potential cost management information has in assisting hospitals to document their financial and market performance.

Mendenhall, S., Shepherd, R., and Kobrinski, E. Cost accounting in healthcare organizations: who needs it? *Healthcare Financial Management* 41(1):34–36, 38, 40, Jan. 1987.

There is no question that improved cost information can lead to improved accountability in health care; however, the major proponents of borrowing cost accounting concepts from manufacturing have not gone far enough. They have ignored an important aspect of manufacturing cost accounting that is also a very important part of hospitals and health care, namely the concern for quality. Within the hospital setting, there are many examples of poor quality that have a direct impact on the cost of providing that service. These include (1) services for the patient that had to be repeated, (2) services not performed for the patient that caused problems, and (3) services performed for the patient that caused problems. Using these three examples, the authors illustrate how a hospital can statistically determine how they can lead to unnecessary costs and substandard quality. Defining these three problems as hospital "rework" (analogous to the manufacturer's "scrap" and "rework"), the authors indicate that the most practical method of capturing and accumulating cost information relating to hospital rework is through the patient accounting system. They discuss three methods that can be used to accumulate this information: write-offs of patient accounts, repeat examination write-offs, and partial write-offs of complications. These transactions could then be summarized for separate reporting through the hospital's case mix system to identify costs associated with quality problems.

Tselepis, J. N. Refined cost accounting produces better information. *Healthcare Financial Management* 43(5):27–28, 32, 34, May 1989.

Cost accounting systems provide management with information crucial to operating more efficiently in today's competitive health care environment. Enhanced cost systems are simple to implement because they parallel existing hospital charge systems. By modifying existing cost systems, health care institutions can generate more accurate cost information necessary for dealing with third-party payers, physicians, and managed care organizations. These articles discuss the required data elements to support a cost accounting system, the methods of gathering cost information, and how to perform a cost analysis.

Decision Support Systems

Brice, J. Decision support. *Healthcare Forum Journal* 32(2):19–21, 24–25, Mar.–Apr. 1989.

Nearly everything relevant to hospital decision support is changing simultaneously. Medicare prospective payment and managed care, in the form of health maintenance organizations (HMOs) and preferred provider organizations (PPOs), are responsible for fundamental changes in the way hospitals are paid. Software technology is also changing rapidly. Executive decision support systems, based upon relational data bases and written in fourth-generation computer languages, are being introduced. Such innovations are making it easier and faster to draw relevant information from various electronic sources in the hospital. This article discusses the use of decision support systems in analyzing managed care contracts. It provides information on the functions of decision support systems with a peripheral examination into their relationship with negotiating managed care contracts. It also describes several new decision support systems in use today. Throughout the article, the author supplies the reader with perspectives from health care managers and researchers regarding the use of decision support systems in the hospital information environment.

Haskell, R. E. Decision support systems: the next step. *Topics in Health Care Financing* 14(2):42–51, Winter 1987.

The new market-driven environment is putting a whole new set of pressures on health care providers. Financing pressures and improvements in technology and medical technique are encouraging a shift from expensive inpatient hospital to ambulatory and other nonacute care environments. Owing to this competitive pressure and the proliferation of nonhospital-owned ambulatory care facilities, providers must learn how to control costs without compromising the quality of care, attract the buyers and consumers of medical care through effective pricing and marketing, assess the impact of offering new or modified services to the community or contracting with managed care plans, and test the viability of alliances or consolidation with other facilities. A good decision support system is needed to meet these challenges. This article explores the role of decision support systems in this competitive environment by addressing and then answering the following questions: "What is . . . ?" "What if . . . ?" and "What next . . . ?" The "what is . . . ?" component is satisfied by an information system; the "what if . . . ?" component is satisfied by modeling systems; and the "what next . . . ?" component is satisfied by expert systems. The author defines and describes each of these systems and provides examples in the form of case studies to illustrate their implementation and use.

Klafehn, K. A., Rakich, J. S., and Kuzdrall, P. J. The use of simulation as an aid in hospital management decision making. *Hospital Topics* 67(2):6–12, Mar.–Apr. 1989.

Changes to the health service delivery environment of the 1980s have forced hospital managers to think differently about their organizations' allocation and use of resources. Simulation, increasingly used as a device for assessing management choices, is the subject of this article. The authors demonstrate its power to assist managers to make better decisions in general and its specific use as a decision-making aid in the assignment of beds among service units. After a brief discussion of the changed environment for hospitals, simulation as a management tool is presented, including a brief literature review of its applications. The simulation mode designed for a 423-bed not-for-profit hospital follows. Finally, the consequences of the reallocation of beds between two service areas, surgery and orthopedics, are graphically presented. Key variables measured include bed utilization, the number of patients awaiting entry to a given service unit, the percentage of patients gaining entry to the service without delay, and the number of patients treated off service.

Malhotra, N. K. Decision support systems for health care marketing managers. *Journal of Health Care Marketing* 9(2):20–28, June 1989.

Health care organizations are encouraged to implement decision support systems geared to meeting the challenges of tomorrow. The author outlines a decision support system (DSS) and illustrates its usefulness for health care marketing managers. A schematic representation of a DSS is described. Applications of DSS in strategic marketing and planning, product, promotion, pricing, and distribution decisions are discussed. Potential problems of integrating DSS into the health care organization are identified, and some useful guidelines for implementation are offered.

Ambulatory Care Data Needs under Prospective Payment

Cohn, D. M., and Shaw, P. L. Development of outpatient databases. *Computers in Healthcare* 9(4):88–89, Apr. 1988.

As more and more hospitals begin to shift some of their services and products to the outpatient sector in response to the revenue crunch imposed by the inpatient prospective payment system (PPS), the federal government noticed a dramatic increase in expenditures for outpatient care. As a result, the federal government has called for the development of a prospective pricing system (PPS) for reimbursing all Medicare outpatient services. The PPS outpatient model should be ready for national implementation by 1991. To ensure maximum reimbursement under outpatient PPS, hospitals will have to submit complete and accurate data to the fiscal intermediaries because these data will be used to determine payment weights. This article provides information on the design and implementation of an outpatient data base. It addresses such issues as the role of the outpatient code editor, data needs, and the importance of the medical record.

Felts, W. R. Classification standards for billing databases and health care reimbursement. *M.D. Computing* 5(2):20–26, 53, Mar.–Apr. 1988.

Third-party payers' demands for demographic information, and for details about symptoms, diagnoses, procedures, and services, are rapidly becoming more complex. Meanwhile, there is a widespread move to standardize the information required on various forms, along with related codes. This standardization could simplify the work of physicians and hospitals. It will permit billing information to be saved in large computer data bases; and the analysis of this information will shape national policies, especially regarding resource utilization and reimbursement. Substantial involvement by health care professionals is needed to ensure that the stored data are complete, consistent, reliable, and properly interpreted. This article describes past and future efforts to develop standardized coding systems for the necessary data (for both inpatient and outpatient encounters)— without unmanageable complexity or oversimplification.

Grimaldi, P. L. Inching toward prospective payment for outpatient hospital care. *Nursing Management* 18(8):26–28, Aug. 1987.

The Health Care Financing Administration (HCFA) has recently revised and expanded the list of ambulatory surgical procedures that Medicare reimburses on a prospective basis. This represents a step toward the federal government's goal of reimbursing all outpatient hospital care at fixed, predetermined rates. To accommodate this change, hospitals must begin to implement operational changes in medical record documentation, billing, and information system requirements. This article provides information regarding proposed changes in ambulatory surgery payment as they affect covered procedures and reimbursement. It also discusses impending changes in the payment system and how they will affect both areas as well. Throughout the article, references are made to the impact these payment system changes will have on the information systems environment.

Koska, M. T. Survey reveals cost, time of PPS conversion. *Hospitals* 63(13):78, July 5, 1989.

A recent survey administered by the American Hospital Association's Society for Ambulatory Care Professionals (SACP) revealed a sampling of what hospitals can expect in terms of changing staffing and management control patterns when outpatient payment is converted into a prospective pricing system. This article summarizes the most important findings of the survey including the effect of the conversion on billing systems, personnel requirements, medical record documentation, and accounts receivable. In addition, it discusses strategies hospitals are employing to address the changes prospective pricing will impose on the information systems environment in ambulatory health care.

Patterson, P. OR directors plan strategies for new outpatient PPS. *OR Manager* 3(12):1, 4, 9, Dec. 1987.

Operating room directors and financial managers are planning strategies for coping with the transition to Medicare prospective payment for hospital-based outpatient surgery. They know that leaner days are ahead. This article outlines those issues operating room managers will have to confront in order to streamline costs and maximize reimbursement. Among the issues discussed are (1) how to organize outpatient surgery services—integrated or freestanding, (2) getting a handle on costs, specifically in the area of cost accounting, (3) unbundling charges, and (4) streamlining nursing practices to control costs.

Sabin, M., and Fox-Gliessman, D. The exploding demand for ambulatory care data. *Computers in Healthcare* 9(6):14–15, 18, June 1988.

Increasing pressures are being placed on members of the health care delivery system to develop a comprehensive, integrated outpatient data base for all outpatient programs. These pressures are most strongly articulated by the federal government in its progress toward a prospective reimbursement system for ambulatory visits. Although there is recognition that large volumes of data exist throughout ambulatory care, these data have limited potential because of their lack of uniformity, clinical/financial integration, and universal availability. This article discusses the work being done to develop a standardized and coordinated ambulatory care data set. It examines and analyzes the Uniform Ambulatory Medical Care Minimum Data Set (UAMCMDS), coding conventions, and outpatient medical record formats. The authors also provide and discuss five issues hospitals must confront when they establish a reliable data-collection system—data verification, cost-effective data transfer, data entry and retrieval, multiplicity of data formats, and external data validity.

The Uniform Ambulatory Care Data Set. *Journal of the American Medical Record Association (AMRA)* 60(10):39–43, Oct. 1989.

The purpose of the Uniform Ambulatory Care Data Set is to improve the comparability of ambulatory care data by defining a common core of standard data items. These items are considered to be those most likely to be needed by a variety of users for multiple applications. Over the years, the integrity and usefulness of the data set have been evaluated, and attempts have been made to refine and expand it to make it more meaningful and statistically relevant. The information in this article was abstracted from the June 1989 report of the National Commission on Vital and Health Statistics (NCVHS) Subcommittee on Ambulatory Care Data Statistics and the Interagency Task Force on the Uniform Ambulatory Care Data Set. The article highlights the following information, which is of importance to the future role and tasks of the ambulatory health care information systems environment: definitions of provider, ambulatory care, and encounter; patient data items; provider data items; and encounter data items. Whereas the 1981 data set defined those items that should be entered in the records of all ambulatory health care, this revision emphasizes that, to the extent possible, these items should be abstracted uniformly from those records into ambulatory care data bases. This brings the data set into accordance with the Uniform Hospital Discharge Data Set and reflects that an increasing number of public- and private-sector groups are recognizing the need for collecting and analyzing data on ambulatory care for a variety of purposes. These purposes include patient care, quality assurance, reimbursement, policy development, management and planning, and research.

Future Trends

Davis, J. A., and Ladd, R. D. Computer aided medicine. *U.S. Healthcare* 6(7):20–22, 24, July 1989.

Initial health care information systems focused on the automation of manual functions. Current systems are becoming increasingly sophisticated. Modern systems utilize local area networks (LANs), relational data bases, fourth-generation languages, end-user computing, physician office integration, voice recognition and integration of data and image, digital imaging, and artificial intelligence. The use of these new technologies is helping to restructure the work environment of the practicing physician. Of extreme interest regarding health care information systems applications is the area of artificial intelligence technology (AIT). This article primarily focuses on the development of AIT, specifically expert systems, and how it will impact the future practice of medicine. The article examines the architecture of an expert system and possible approaches that can be used to design an expert system's knowledge base. It also provides a listing and description of expert systems in use today, including AI/RHEUM (rheumatology), HEADMED (psychopharmacology), ONCOCIN (cancer), and PIP (renal diseases), to name a few. All of the expert systems discussed in the article have been designed to aid the physician in making decisions. Their development and use will continue to increase as acceptance is gained by physicians.

Hume, S. The hospital of the here and now. *Health Progress* 70(10);55–58, 70, Oct. 1989.

In the future, it will be imperative that new hospital information systems provide real benefits. However, benefits will become a bigger issue as information systems compete with "bricks and mortar" and new clinical services for fewer available dollars. This article examines the deficiencies in hospital information systems as they exist today and then proceeds to examine the future information needs of health care providers. It analyzes and summarizes a variety of arguments concerning user demands, systems communication, integration versus interface, and the intelligent network and how these relate to the information systems environment of the future. According to the author, the ultimate solution is the intelligent network. In an intelligent network, the system manages all the components in terms of knowing what data are where; and it knows whenever it gets an update what data base needs to be updated. It does integrity checking to make sure the data bases are synchronized; it controls all the communications, security, backup, and recovery functions; and it also does the presentation management. The article also briefly discusses other future offerings in the communications field besides intelligent networking.

McConnell, D. H., and Brenner, M. A. HIS: the clinician's role. *Computers in Healthcare* 10(6):20–22, 24, June 1989.

The technology transition in health care is being fueled by three major forces: new demand, new users, and new technology. Although hospital information systems are in the midst of the technological revolution in health care, many clinicians believe that present-day hospital information systems have been largely ineffective. Little automation of the medical and nursing information management process actually exists in most systems. Those areas where computer assistance does exist usually consist of a single niche, such as order communications or results reporting. The author points out that in more full-functioned systems the major problem areas can best be described as unnatural access codes (constrained by computer menu hierarchy) and lack of information integration. The article concludes with a discussion of these problem areas and how future information systems can be redesigned to accommodate the specific needs of the physicians, nurses, and other allied health personnel. In the conclusion, the author points out that if future information systems are to meet the divergent needs of health care practitioners, workstation technology will have to be adopted.

Pearce, D. Key executives speak out. *Computers in Healthcare* 8(8):26–27, 29, 31, 33–35, Aug. 1987.

Is top management concerned with health care information needs? Given the recent rise of the position of chief information officer (CIO) and the common belief that top managers in health care are still largely computer-shy, how would top health care executives respond to a request to describe their current and future information needs? In developing this article, a dozen executives were contacted. Despite their overbooked schedules, nine were eager to make their information needs known, two referred to other persons within the organization, and one declined an interview. This response indicated the high level of concern that chief executives have for information. Although the original intent of this article was to focus on the decision support needs of chief executives and chief operating officers, those interviewed were very vocal about their additional needs in several areas. These included the need to (1) model future management information systems to coincide with their vision of the future health care system model, (2) share information between physician practices and their organizations, and (3) provide shared data bases of noncompetitive information among health care providers and between providers and insurance carriers to ease the costs and financial risks of admissions, billing, and insurance verification.

Toole, J., and Campbell, S. HL7: the systems integration opportunity. *U.S. Healthcare* 6(7):14, 16, July 1989.

Currently, a group of hospitals, system vendors, and consultants are working to establish a communication protocol called the HL7 Project. The HL7 Project will establish a standard communication protocol, message format, and definition of data elements at the application layer to facilitate communication between dissimilar hardware and software health care systems. When a system communicates with other systems, the messages will adhere to predetermined standards. This will greatly reduce the cost of interfacing. This article summarizes the history behind the HL7 Project, the reasoning behind its creation, and its impact on the future status of health care information processing.

Ummel, S. L. HIS—an elusive promise in troubled times: a CEO's view. *Computers in Healthcare* 10(6):65–66, 68, June 1989.

Hospitals and information technology stand at a potentially exciting and yet perplexing juncture today. Both industries are caught in major economic transformations, and this common force may dictate how they interrelate and shape each other's longer-term destinies. The state of hospital information systems, from a comparative technological and performance standpoint, is a lingering disappointment to most hospital executives. Many hospitals are poised for significant investment in new or replacement computer systems. However, their deteriorating financial results, coupled with limited and unreliable computer products, may distance one of the nation's largest industries further behind their service counterparts in cost-effective information technology. This article examines the future relationship between the hospital and information technology industries.

The author discusses such issues as the hospital culture and how it may affect the implementation of information systems; the relationship between hospitals and computer vendors; and future marketplace developments in information technology.

Vendors predict growth in ambulatory care software. *Hospitals* 61(15):96, 98, Aug. 5, 1987.

Many health care managers agree that software devoted to the ambulatory side of the health care equation will grow in the future. Although health maintenance organizations (HMOs) and preferred provider arrangements (PPAs) are presently interested only in "basic and fundamental" software applications such as appointment scheduling and billing systems, their interest in packages that address quality of care review, utilization review, and financial management will increase over the coming years. This article provides a concise perspective on the changing marketplace for ambulatory care software. It discusses vendor applications as well as those developed in-house.